COURAGEOUS CAREGIVER

Support, encouragement, and tools to aid our heroes who partake in home healthcare for those with dementia.

CURTIS L WALKER

Courageous Caregiver

Copyright © 2015

ISBN: 978-0-9971168-0-9

*Dedicated to my family and the thriving bond
that we share.*

The Caregiver Commitment

LIVE ❖ *LOVE* ❖ *LEAVE*

*As a caregiver, I commit to **LIVE** my life at its highest level and to make sure I show up for it every day and in every way.*

*I commit to **LOVE** everyone that is placed in front of me and find a way to love what I am doing in full joy.*

*I commit to live my life in such a way that it becomes legendary and contagious and I **LEAVE** a legacy that shapes the world I live in because I simply chose to stand up and do something about it.*

In honor and loving memory of
❖Annette Walker❖
My dear sister, a mother, and a friend to so many.

My inspiration for this book.
My eternal dreamer.

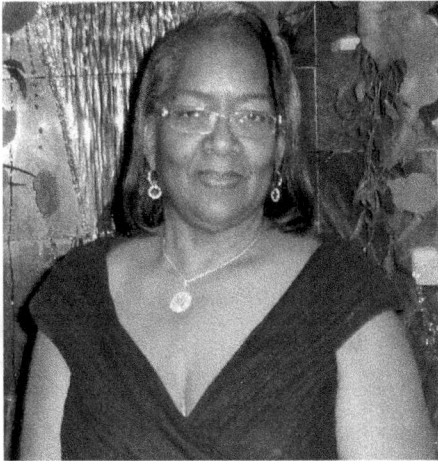

Born:
March 25, 1954

Ascended to heaven:
June 7, 2015

Table of Contents

Prologue

"God, grant me the serenity to accept the things I cannot change, the courage to change the things I can, and the wisdom to know the difference" – Reinhold Niebuhr

You picked up this book because something about this title piqued your interest. You may be asking yourself what a "courageous caregiver" actually *is*. More than likely, if you find yourself reading this book, you or someone you know is engaged in some level of care for a loved one. You may have experienced the physical, mental and emotional effects that follow that responsibility. It's estimated that 1 out of every 5 families in the United States is involved in some form of direct care. Within 10 years, 1 out of 2 families will be impacted. The numbers are overwhelming. What's getting done about this? It seems hopeless. Good thing I am not of that school of thought. It is my purpose through this book and this movement to give you hope and to equip you with the tools to enable you to say "YES." Yes, you can do something about what has happened to you. Yes, you can do something about what has happened to your loved one. Yes, you can still have love and live. Yes, you can have hope for a brighter tomorrow. If you can hang with me through this journey, I promise you that I will show you a glimmer of hope.

What's Going On?

"The secret to change is to focus all of your energy not on fighting the old, but on building the new" – **Socrates**

Most of this book is dedicated to the work I had to engage in personally as I cared for my older sister as she battled dementia. When I began this care process, I was in way over my head. The disease was not something we could foresee or could logically prepare for. With this book, my intent is to equip you with some practical working knowledge that will aid you in your day-to-day task of caring.

Without an understanding of what you are facing, you will be forced to manage your situation blind, and it will come with the strength and shock of a tsunami. Many uninformed and unprepared caregivers have submitted blindly to the seemingly sole option of using heavy medication to address the mental state and care of their loved one, and in some cases themselves. In providing care, there are many obstacles to consider that cannot be remedied with the "quick fix" of medication.

Some of the issues I had to address where:
Getting a proper diagnosis
Understanding the implications and prognosis of that diagnosis
Organizing help from family and friends
Scheduling support
Addressing healthcare cost
Getting financial support
Addressing legal issues
Dealing with personal health and mental well-being
Considering the impact on family dynamics and job responsibilities

In the upcoming chapters, I will give you help, support and a strategy on how to address some critical issues, and I will also set you up with resources that could further assist you.

The Short Story

"If we are growing, we're always going to be out of our comfort zone." – John C Maxwell

I was blind-sided by this disease, and I initially fought against it, which in turn caused me to fight against my sister, Annette. Because I was not yet equipped to deal with all that I would face, my actions created a riff in the family. It was a huge undertaking trying to understand where this disease would eventually lead. It was difficult coordinating medical and family help. It was a blow to my faith because I had been, and still am, researching a cure for the disease. I know and feel in my heart that a cure is on its way, but it will come too late for my sister. I did, however, get lucky by finding a wonderful adult daycare. The workers helped me understand the realities of dementia, and they gave me a better perspective on what to expect. Still, I was determined not to let this disease overpower the essence of my sister or destroy our family. I was not going to let it put me in a place where I could not be the best for myself and for my family. The tools I found along my journey enabled me to deal with the disease with power and love.

I received one of the best gifts of all. I discovered who I was through all of this. I found out how strong I am. I saw images of real unconditional love. And most importantly, I learned that when taking care of someone else, it is imperative that I never neglect myself. Two extremes can exist when providing care for someone else: self-centeredness can occur when you resent your loved one and, on the other side, it is possible to neglect your own personal health in favor of your loved one's quality of life. I had to talk to a lot of families and health care professionals to get a balanced perspective on this matter.

Overall, I had to grasp the concept of balance and hope in the middle of a complicated situation. As you continue through this caregiving manual, you will find that you are able to tap into the incredible network of people that are out there, people who are ready, willing, and able to help you. I have seen some people overlook the help, and I have seen the physical and emotional trauma that care has left on the caregiver. I have seen cases of caregiving that have led to the caregiver's death. In some instances, the stress has even led to suicide or homicide. I want to give reassurance that it does not have to come to that. There is a way, and there's help. Be patient. Read the chapters. Take good notes. And by all means, go to our interactive website and connect with the many others that are out there and get the help you desperately need. There is strength in the community.

As you experience my writings, I want to give you the gift of hope. I received hope in my journey. Back when I began this journey, I was a bitter and beaten person. I felt down and guilty. I felt loaded with remorse, pain, and no sense of hope. I lost my cause and real desire to celebrate life. I wasn't living; I was going through the motions and just merely existing. I hope my experience helps you. If you are feeling hopeless and down, it is my desire that through this writing you find means to feel alive again. I pray you can move past the many levels of grief and walk in a realm of wholeness.

Why Read this Book?

"The test of a civilization is in the way that it cares for its helpless members." – Pearl S Buck

The knowledge researchers have gained when it comes to dementia has been coming faster than the rate of trying to get a sip from a water hose. 90% of what we know comes from studies conducted within the past 15 years. Along with developing medications, there are techniques to aid you in your care, while at the same time preserving your loved one's dignity and enhancing your relationship. If you can use this guide and put in the time, you will be well equipped to promote care for your loved one in a harmonious environment that can support the highest level of health that can exist within the confines of this disease.

I will not sugar coat this and say that it will be easy. There are days when your loved one will be emotionally off the charts. This care will physically and emotionally task you and challenge even the calmest of individuals to lose their cool. But, by being equipped, you will have the means to face the disease with wisdom, strength, strategy, dignity, and love. My intent is to provide you with tools and to get you plugged into a network of support. You are not alone.

If you have been caring for a loved one for quite some time, it is possible that a dark shadow has fallen over the life you lived before the disease. It would appear that your former life got wiped away. Please, allow me to speak to the bruised soul inside of you. I want to encourage you to not let go of the person you were or the goals you had; I want you to wait before you put them in the grave.

You see, there are many books out there on how to provide care, but there are not many on how a caregiver should care for themselves. This may feel like a foreign concept. You may be saying, "How in the world can I take care of my mom and still have time to work my full-time job?" I can sympathize with that concern. My job was put at risk while I was taking care of my sister, and I eventually found myself unemployed. Still, I can tell you that there is hope. I just had to do a hard paradigm shift in my thinking to see how to balance things in a healthy way for all that were involved.

This book will challenge you and push your thinking to the limit. It will give you some action steps. If you move on it, you can experience some tremendous results. Much of what I learned came through trial and error, but I also consulted professionals in the field. As you work through this process, I would love to hear from you. Please visit *CourageousCaregiver.org* and look for the feedback option. It will help me with any enhancements I may need to make to my later editions.

Chapter 1 – Our Story

Where we stand

"Being challenged in life is inevitable, being defeated is optional." - Unknown

According to the Alzheimer's Association, there are 5 million people in the US with dementia and that number is projected to be 7 million by the end of 2015. 1 out of every 5 families in the US has felt tasked with caring for a loved one with dementia or Alzheimer's, and within the next 10 years that number will climb to 1 out of every 2 families. With those alarming numbers, caregivers are facing burnout, depression, and hopelessness. Many feel isolated, beaten and broken. Some feel ill-equipped for the task at hand. I've been there. I have felt the pain. I have stared into the face of death, and I saw my own. I was in way over my head, and I needed help. I started with prayer. Prayer led me to actionable steps that enabled me to cut through a lot of red tape and develop a deeper understanding of what I was up against from a physical, financial, mental, emotional and spiritual point of view. I have had to look at this thing from all angles. I've engaged in helping other families, and through that engagement, the idea for this book was conceived. My aim is to aid you and to give you resources to develop a community in order to promote the highest level of health and hope for the heroic caregiver in you.

I entitled this book *Courageous Caregiver* because it takes a great deal of courage to do what you do, day in and day out. I define courage as knowing that there is danger ahead, but you still keep moving forward. In some cases, that may be interpreted as crazy, but in reality it takes a little bit of that to do the job, and if you are not crazy going in, you may be going out.

How things have changed

"Change the changeable, accept the unchangeable, and remove yourself from the unacceptable." - Unknown

When I started this process, I was like a fish out of the water. I did not have a clue where to turn. I did not know who to turn to for advice. I was in denial about the disease, and that prevented me from asking for the right kind of help. There were not many resources out there that addressed the emotional needs of a caregiver. So, my goal is to provide you with a comprehensive resource that you can easily turn to and from which you can pull some great references and strategies.

To be honest, what I am proposing is not an easy topic to address. If you are knee deep in the care process, it is extremely hard to take the time to lift your head and look up. Unless you are a naturally motivated and driven person, some of the concepts I will bring up may seem heavy. But trust me, I had to realign my focus and practices to be a healthier me while providing quality care.

When I looked at my sister's situation and the changes she was going through, I allowed my life, health, emotions, and outlook on life to get entangled with the disease, and I lost my way for a moment. I felt helpless and hopeless. I was bitter at her and what this disease had made of her life as well as what it was doing to my own life.

It took help from some loving friends that taught me to value my health highly. It took a community of other, like-minded, caring people to help me see the value and importance of what I was doing. I had to value myself enough to not play the victim roll. I naturally had to work on addressing the needs of my loved one, but I also had to make sure I had the correct perspective of health for the both of us. My focus had to be on her having life to the fullest capacity that she could handle based on what the disease was offering for that given day. I did all of this while at the same time hoping, working, and developing the life that I wanted. I always had to make sure that there was time put in toward investing in myself and showing myself just as much love. I had to learn not to play the blame game for the disease or how bad I think my life may have been at the moment. I had to allow myself to see that events happen in season and that my life was not going to stay stuck in hardship for eternity. I had to learn to watch what those seasons were and to adjust to make the best of every season and to draw the best that I can at every turn.

Now, the bad news
"Life is like photography.   You need negatives to develop." - Unknown
Now let me make this clear. I am not a doctor, and I do not have a bunch of fancy letters behind my name. I do have a degree, but that is in Information Technology. I have never worked in a nursing home, but I have spent hundreds of hours in hospitals, nursing homes, and care facilities with family and friends that I have had to provide care for over the years. I come from

a large family, and I have lived in a loving environment. I have also traveled the world and have seen the results of how bad diseases can impact the human body, and I have also seen how horrible one human can be to another. I have seen people go through some incredible lengths to find help and peace for their loved ones, and I have seen a lot of despair when it comes to not finding the right answers. I know what it is to feel the misery of knowing your loved one has an incurable disease. I have a clear view of the contrast. I care about humanity and the direction we are headed. I know I am not offering a cure for the disease, but I commit my full engagement in helping those who are. However, in the meantime, my pressing desire is how we function until the cures development. I understand the value of having high hope while faced with insurmountable odds. I want to encourage you to have and develop a perseverant attitude. It does not seem fair that you have to watch the person you love, and may have cared for you at an earlier time, go through so much, and you have to pick up the pieces and go on with life. But, I have to lay this one important reason to care for someone before you. HONOR! I want to honor the life and memory of my sister. I want to honor her values. My sister, before this disease hit, was a person that pursued life. She lived it at its highest level. If she were in her right mind and had to take a look at how I was living when I was at my low point, she would say, "You are not doing me any favors by feeling the way you feel. Your feelings are not going to bring me back. But you can at least honor my memory by living your life to the fullest." In this book, I want to offer you the essence of her heart.

LIVE! Live life to the fullest. LIVE WITH NO REGRETS.

New approach

"You must learn a new way to think before you can master a new way to be" – Marianne Williamson

Allow me to distinguish your role as *home* caregiver vs. the role of a nursing home. First of all, to set the record straight, not all nursing homes are bad, evil, or a dark place where your loved ones go to die. There are some wonderful places out there that do a phenomenal job of meeting the needs of the residents. There are some smiling faces that have some of the best training to know how to love on and connect with your loved one. They ensure treatment with dignity and respect. I am not ignoring the fact there are some horror stories of some bad places, but I am of the mindset that your personal level of research and involvement manages much of the success of a nursing home experience. I will get into that in later chapters, plus I have another book coming out to address that in detail. Keep a watch out for that.

But, I said all that to get to my main point: there is no one who can care for your loved one better than you. You have a committed investment. You have blood, heart, and soul connections all wrapped up with the care you are providing. For you, it is not a day-to-day job. It is a way of life. It is a labor of love. It is you, living by your faith, in many cases. Honoring your core beliefs, you are placed in a position where you have to take on the role of detective, nurse, lawyer, referee, psychologist, priest, exorcist, police officer, and so much more. Each roll changes daily. After going for a prolonged period, you get worn out and stressed to the max. Some have made the mistake of trying to play the superhero and try to be the catch all/end all to meet every need of their loved one. Trust me when I say that this can be one of the costliest and unhealthiest mistakes you, as a caregiver, could ever make. I know this is hard to face, especially if that person is your spouse.

I spent time with some dear friends; I will call them Joe and Connie, for the sake of this print. Joe was 70, and Connie was slightly younger, and they had been married for 40 plus years. Connie had been ill for a very long time and had to go into the hospital for cardiopulmonary issues. Joe was right by her side. It was amazing watching them interact daily. After being in the hospital for quite some time, the insurance company moved Connie to a nursing home. Joe was there early every morning and stayed by her side till late at night. Connie's condition made her, at times, a very difficult person to be around, and she would forget who she was, where she was, who was caring for her, and how bad her condition was. Joe loved Connie so much that he would open himself up to her abuse brought on by her illness. After talking to Joe about his situation, I came to find out that six months earlier Joe had to get a triple by-pass operation. He fought to recover and as a part of his therapy he had to practice deliberate relaxation techniques. It amazed me to watch how calm Joe could keep himself as Connie unleashed her tirades upon him. I bring this up to highlight for couples—you are committed to love, in sickness and health, and till death do you part. That being said, there has to be a healthy boundary you establish for how deep you are going to let the disease dig into your heart vs. how deep you are going to let true love dig.

One thing I can say for certain, if I had to face this all over again, two areas I would have adjusted in my life right out of the gate were educating myself in the area of communicating with a person with dementia and seeking out and organizing helpful resources up front. Those steps would have made a world of difference with addressing some of the tense situations that developed. The first inclination is to get the patient on all sorts of medications, but if you are going to take that approach, it is inadvisable to take a pill for every little thing that a person is experiencing. Each pill you introduce creates another set of problems that you have to get another pill to address. If you get too many combinations, you reduce the quality of life. My goal is to help you understand the phases of the disease so that you can better manage your responses to your loved one. This will in turn give you a more relatable time with your loved one and can lead to less stress for you and for them as you work through the progressive stage of this disease.

Of all the minds that you have to protect throughout every stage of the disease, yours is the most important. As a caregiver, you have to be deliberate about protecting your physical health. You also have to put in time to protect and enhance your mental health. I have seen many caregivers lose so much of themselves in the care of their loved ones that they neglect to fight for their own value, nor do they feel that they deserve to have a future since their loved one seemingly cannot have one. I have also seen instances where they resent their loved one because of what the disease has done to their life and how it has become so draining.

It took a lot of balanced perspective as well as focused faith development to help me through my process. I will introduce you to a few different techniques that will prove to be invaluable as you walk through the chapters. Not every case is the same. There are over 80 types of dementia, and each case, combined with other medical factors, can lead to a wide variety of approaches. However, there are some common patterns, and my research has rooted much of that out, and I have developed a good strategy to address the care of the person with the disease, as well as the caregiver themselves.

How I figured it all out

"The formulation of a problem is often more essential than its solution, which may be merely a matter of mathematics or experimental skills." – Albert Einstein

I got dropped into this jungle firefight and had to figure it out as I went along. I had plenty of people say they would pray for me, but that carried little weight when it came to making a real difference. I sought advice and much of it came from people who did not have an understanding of what my sister was going through nor did they even have a clue what I was feeling. I had a hard time telling people about how I felt because it often came across that they really did not care. Either they would change the subject or the look on their face was that of pure disinterest. That was a period of my life, where I felt alone, isolated, and misunderstood. As you read, much of the flow will be like a timeline of what I had to face while caring for my sister, beginning with her life before the disease and leading into how and when we first found out. I will talk about her care and coordination and the support we received, and finally I will take you on the journey of hospice care. Much of what I learned came through trial and error as well as seeking help from some wonderful professionals. A lot of the information existed in scattered form in many locations, so I made it my goal and commitment to bring it all together and put all under one roof.

Who wins? - Who loses?

"Yesterday is not ours to recover, but tomorrow is ours to win or lose." – Lyndon B. Johnson

When you care for a person with dementia, you can practically take ten years off your life. This book will help you fight back and come out as a winner. That is a bold claim, but it is true and possible by implementing these actionable steps. This book will give you a framework approach on how to view certain situations and how to address them, so that they create minimal damage to yourself, your family, and the loved one under your care.

To take this book and to stop reading at this point, may add pain and heartache to your care plans for your loved one. I am invested and committed to helping every caregiver feel equipped to give the best care and to care equally for themselves. In many cases, a caregiver gets so emotionally invested that they overlook some key issues that will impact them personally and will impact the person under their care. Use this book to help you prepare and respond. Also, if you know of someone facing this issue, please, by all means, buy a copy and send it to him or her. Before you send it to them, please have them visit *CourageousCaregiver.org.* and check out the welcome video.

It is of deep concern to me when I witness caregivers experience a nervous breakdown while under the strain of caregiving. I pray and fight for each of you. My heart goes out to you and what you are experiencing. I value each and every one of you. I walk with you as you grieve the daily loss of your loved one. I speak to the soul of the one who feels bruised and in many cases abandoned, isolated, and neglected. I want to remind you that, above and beyond popular belief, you are not alone. It took a lot of heart to stand up and do what you have done. You had the option to walk away, but you chose to jump into the fight. You chose to love. People have indicated on many occasions that all the work I had put into taking care of my sister would bless me. It took a little while for it to sink in, but I was already blessed by simply making the choice to help. That choice moved my heart to a higher level. I knew I was valuing human life and had increased my personal value as a human. I felt like I was also connecting with my Creator and the Lover of my soul by choosing to nurture a relation with my sister, who could no longer care for herself. I felt alive and refreshed each time I reached out and met her needs. I learned how to tap into my most valuable strength. I moved from stress and depression into a life of liberty, freedom, and joy. By faith, I was taught that I carry the light of my heavenly kingdom wherever I go. So, each time I interacted with my sister, I got to bring the presence of God into her chaos and brought order and peace to her madness. I feel blessed and delighted to serve and it is my aim, through this reading, to stir your heart to also be inspired, and to help you feel blessed and empowered.

❖Chapter 1 – Our Story❖

❖Chapter 1 – Our Story❖

Chapter 2 – Help in the Time of Trouble
More of our story

"You either walk inside your story and own it, or you stand outside your story and hustle for your worthiness." – Brene Brown

Before we jump into the disease and the care, to give you a good view of the situation, I have to tell you about myself. I was born in the city of Pontiac, Michigan back in 1965. Back then, the economy was still booming. I was the youngest of seven. I had six older sisters (one of whom passed away before I was born) and an older brother. The sibling that was closest to my age was six years older than me, my sister Ora. All of my sisters were loving to me, but also very tough on me. It was as if I had six mothers watching over me. My sister Annette, whom I will talk about more in later chapters of this book, was a middle child. She is approximately 12 years older than me. When she was not working, she was my main babysitter. I have some fond memories of her in my growing up years. I remember back in the early seventies when she taught me how to navigate the routes of city bus mass transportation. She would take me to downtown Pontiac which was, during that time, the happening place.

Those were extraordinary times. It was great being a kid during those times. My family comes from a southern heritage. They migrated to Pontiac, Michigan in the early 1960's because of the automotive boom. Our father, James Walker, worked in the Pontiac Motors metal foundry. He was a hardworking man. Our mother, Jessie Walker (Hooper), was a high-spirited and God-fearing woman. She was a no-nonsense kind of lady, and she raised her kids to have respect for herself and other. We were a close family. There were times where we got a little rough with each other, but no matter what, I always felt loved.

One thing I admired about all of my sisters was that they were all hard workers like our mom. They all adopted a strong faith and learned to believe in God and to believe in themselves as much as God believed in them as well. I want to highlight my sister Annette in this segment since most of this is about the transitions she had to go through.

Annette, early on, worked in jobs where she could care for people. She loved connecting and relating to people. She was very ambitious. After high school, because of limited funds, she could not attend college, but she was dedicated and went to work every day. Oakland County employed her for the WIC (Women Infant Children) department. Her job was to work with young single mothers to ensure they had a healthy baby. She managed the immunization department. She did not stop there, because the older she got, the more ambitious she got.

She started her family early on. She was a mother of three by the age of 26. She never married, but had a strong desire to do so. Even though she never married, she did not allow that to set her back in providing for her children, nor did she let that diminish her drive and passion for life. She went through religious training and became a licensed minister. She also started a seamstress business where she designed and made her custom women clothing. She held fashion shows in Pontiac and Detroit. She also worked hard and got a real estate license and worked diligently at selling homes to her clients. At the age of 45, she decided it was time to fight for completion and went to college. At the age of 48, she completed her Bachelor's degree in Business Management at the University of Phoenix. She wanted those skilled to help her move and advance her business.

She was a remarkable lady and unyielding in her expression of love. After watching her life, and looking at her many accomplishments, she served as motivation for me to step up and become more as well. She inspired me to go back to college after I had dropped out so many years earlier. I went back at age 38 and graduated from the University of Phoenix by the time I was 40. Shortly after that, Annette came to me and gave me a book on whose cover she had inscribed, "It's time for you to take it to the next level." The book was a real estate book. She encouraged me to get into buying real estate property. I appreciated the push.

Shortly after that, things got a little heavy physically, mentally and emotionally for Annette and for the rest of her family. When Annette was in her early 50's, she got word that her youngest son, Sedrick fell ill and had been transported to emergency with a brain aneurysm. The doctors were able to catch it in time, but the event took a deep emotional toll on her. Annette was at the hospital every day, and she was under a lot of stress. Because of the stress, it brought on some of the early signs of dementia. She forgot important appointments and the daily tasks she would frequently perform.

Much of the forgetfulness started spilling over into her job, and that was a catalyst that brought the disease to light. She started forgetting critical parts of her job. Her manager insisted that the get checked out and eventually placed her on medical leave. My sister went to the doctor and got the first diagnosis of the disease, but she was in complete denial of what the doctor had revealed to her. She initially tried to handle the effects of the disease on her own. However, as time went on, she was slowly turning her physical, mental, and financial life into a disaster.

One day, I went to apply for credit and was denied. I was shocked by the event, because when I last checked, my credit scores were in the high 700's, but they were then reading down around 350. I was stunned at what I saw, so I looked deeper into the cause. My mother had lived in a house until she passed away in 2014, at which point I became the owner, and I refinanced the mortgage. I worked out a deal with my sister, Annette, to partner with me to take over the mortgage after a season of payments. Before that time, Annette lived with my mother and cared for her until the day she passed away. This business agreement was supposed to be a win-win situation for both of us. She managed all the payments for the mortgage, so I had no reason to check on that matter, however, when the disease hit, she lost sight of how she was managing her payments.   When she got late notices, she was embarrassed and hid all the bills and shut-off notices and foreclosure letters. This had gone on for five months. So, by the time I got involved, the home was going through a foreclosure process.

I was furious and devastated once I found out. When I questioned my sister about the matter, she was extremely defensive and in denial over the entire issue. After asking enough questions, I finally got the clue that there was a medical issue we were addressing. I found out that she was not going to her doctor's appointments, nor was she taking her medication that was to help slow down the effects of the disease.   From that point forward, I had to take an active role in her care.

I, along with her daughter, developed a plan to set up care for her. It was a hard transition for everyone, and we experienced everything imaginable that this disease could throw at a person. Now, I had to admit, I initially handled much of this poorly. I was sympathetic to what she had to go through, but I was furious because of the disruption this was doing to my life. I was working hard and advancing my career and helping my kids graduate from high school and trying to keep peace at home with my wife, not to mention I had a mountain of debt that I was attempting to address. My sister's situation just created one more thing to add to my list. The arrangement I made with my sister's daughter was for her to manage the primary responsibilities for the day-to-day activity and I would assist. Because my sister tried to handle the disease on her own early on— and in such a poor way—it accelerated her symptoms. We had to get the assistance of an adult day care service so that my niece and I would have means to perform our day-to-day work and still provide quality care for my sister.

I would never have imagined, in a million years, that I would be caught up with providing care for anyone in this manner. Caregiving is an enormous stretch for me. At the age of 17 I went away and joined the US Marines. I was trained by some of the best to be the best. I was a focused and driven person. I lived hard, I played hard, and I fought hard. My life did not lend for sensitivity, softness, slowness or gentleness. So early on, when I got pulled into this, my personality strongly clashed with what my sister was experiencing. I was a person with an agenda. When I encountered my sister in this state, it was very frustrating for both of us because she was genuinely confused and had a growing sense of insecurity every day. When I requested for her to perform a simple task, such as putting her shoes on to go outside, it just made her angry and caused her to lash out at everyone around her. My sister even developed a growing hatred for her daughter. Since they lived together in a small house, there were clashes every day, and I was regularly called in to intervene.

One of the challenges I had to face, which I resisted early on, was not willfully adjusting my attitude and life to manage the changing dynamics that this disease would take my entire family through. If I knew back then what I know today, I would have had the means, inner drive, and passion for saying, "I am not in a battle to beat this disease." My real battle was more in line to fight for dignity and wholeness. This disease had peaks and valleys, and I had to equip myself to handle the terrain. I had to become aware of the emotional and psychological shift with the person under my care. I had to improve on how I was managing the transition to promote the highest level of emotional and spiritual health for my loved one as well as myself. I had to develop enough to allow myself to let go of the "traditional" life agenda. I had to be attuned to the disorder and wrong messages that my loved one's brain was telling her and know how to relate to the confusion and promote an atmosphere of comfort and peace. I had to learn to push pride aside and ask for help. There were things lost that I will never get back because of how I handled things related to helping my sister. But, because of this experience and my own personal growth, I clearly know I have gained a much more valuable treasure.

During this long process of care, my focus as well as my job performance diminished. As a result, there was a season when my company had to let me go. I was off work for nine long months, and I was devastated by this loss. As you read this book, I will impart to you some insight that may help address some issues when it comes to the caregiver and their job. If you do not have a good plan going in, you could seriously put your livelihood at risk. The loss could also damage the love and compassion you need to care for your loved one. If not quickly addressed, your feelings could boil over into resentment.

When it came to my sister and my initial manner in dealing with this disease, I did a poor job of understanding the ranges of emotions that that defined her reality. As a Marine, I was conditioned to function in a near flat state, while getting my job done. With my sister, she had every emotion under the sun coming out of her and in no particular order. She would be happy one moment, and then become extremely brutal with the words that would fly out of her mouth. One of the side effects of the disease is that the portion of your brain that controls your discretion is one of the first parts to go. So there was no filter on my sister's mouth, and everything that she had ever heard or experienced would flood out of her mouth with no restraint. Her mind would play tricks on her, and she would become so paranoid about things she had misplaced. There were countless times where she would accuse people of stealing from her. That was the only logical conclusion her mind could come up with. She even went as far as wondering off to the police station and accusing her daughter of stealing food from her. I had to learn some creative techniques to help me address those events while trying to maintain a level of love and respect between the two of us.

Based on how dementia is diagnosed, treated, and monitored, you could potentially get some good years with your loved one. However, the cold hard truth is that dementia ultimately leads to brain death. That was a hard thing for me to face. I worked actively with my sister and this disease for six years. I worked hard with her doctors and neurologist to establish a good quality of life for her, and I also did a lot of research to see if we were getting any close with a cure for what we are dealing with. At the end of each day, I was led back to the same conclusion: it was only a matter of time before the disease would take her mind and her life along with it. This disease would get her to a place, physically, where it would be beyond my limited ability to meet her medical needs. To me, that felt like giving up, and I am not the type of person to handle losing well.

This disease enabled me to work with some great organizations and a wide variety of individuals who love and care for those with dementia. For those who have stepped up to the plate and reached out to care, it is a very noble thing. There are those who are in it just for a paycheck, but there are those that are very passionate about giving loving care to their loved ones that they serve. When it came time for me to make the decision to place my sister in a nursing home, it was a very hard and emotional transition I had to make. I had heard so many horror stories about what goes on in nursing homes. How could I place her in one of those places? It was my given responsibility to watch over her and care for her. I struggled with making the decision. By the time I made the decision, it was way too late. Her condition had progressed so fast that the help she needed I could no longer provide, and I was making her health worse by delaying placing her in a nursing home.

My care for her started to take its toll on my body as well as my mind. I was constantly on the go because of things related to her. Plus, I still had my day job. The mental stress was affecting my relationship with my wife and other family members. Because I made my sister such a high priority, it became difficult for me to manage healthy, active relationships with family and friends. There was an air of mild depression that hung over me. I lost a lot of personal time because of all of this, so I stopped working out on a regular basis, which caused a lot of weight gain. Because I was functioning with the extra weight and reduced muscle strength, I was subject to getting a back injury, which put me out of commission for about a month. I placed myself in a desperate situation. If it was not for the aid of my wife and a couple of my other sisters, I do not think I would have survived.

When I got to the point of considering moving my sister into a nursing home, I battled issues of feeling like I was betraying my sister. But as I walked through the process and sought out good council, I found that I was betraying her more by keeping her with me. I tried to do something I was not equipped to do, and I was sacrificing the stability of my family and extended support group the longer I tried to exercise pride and hang onto something that I was not meant to hold.

This journey was hard and challenging, but it has proven to be beneficial. I had to face some tough decisions, and I had to grow as a part of the process. Because I was facing something that I was somewhat powerless to fix, I had to adjust my views and actions. I initially looked at it as a situation of loss. Each successive day, I felt broken because I knew I would lose pieces of my sister. Statistically, I knew that this could linger on for about ten years or more. That amount of time can lead to two choices: it will either break a person, or it can move you to a place of prayer. I knew that I did not want to get bitter, so I had to find a way to get better. One of the empowering elements I wish to bring to you as you read this is to help you feel and know that it is all right and vital for you to put balance into your life. What I have witnessed is some caregivers either put too much emphasis on the loved one and by doing so, destroy other elements of their life, or they put way too much emphasis on themselves and create an environment of stress, resentment, and abuse. What I am proposing is a lifestyle shift that promotes a high level of respect, love, honor, and dignity for all. As we get further into the pages, I will draw much of this out. I want to thank you for hanging with me so far. I want you to know that I passionately want to see people around me do better. If I have something that I can share to make life a little easier, I will gladly pass it out. I hope this book gives you hope and inspires you. I want to see lives get better and for you to experience tremendous transformation in how you approach this disease as well as life.

❖Chapter 2 – Help in the Time of Trouble❖

I can tell you, what I am going to reveal in this book will not be easy to grasp for some. But I can tell you if an old Marine can experience a life-transforming shift in thought, I know that practically anyone can do this. Another key thing I want you to walk away with from this book are the tools that empower you to have a healthy, thriving relationship with your loved one, no matter what stage they are in with their disease. Some of what I will share will also enhance relationships with others in your circle. Above all, my goal is to get your spirit inspired so you can feel charged and encouraged. I want you to feel good about yourself and do what it takes to protect and enhance your personal health while you care for others in your life.

As you go through this book, there is one important element that I want you to see scattered throughout. I want you to become passionate about building a good team. Some of you may think that you do not have a right to ask for help. Or that you do not know how to ask for help or who to get help from at all. Well, relax. I will show you how. You are not alone. There are people out there who care. Based on how you ask and what you ask them to do will determine how much help you can get and the frequency. You will see that help you request can bring value and life into your dark moments you ultimately will face with this disease. I will show you how to get help from family and friends. I will show you how to draw in new friends that will enable you to experience peace and success when it comes to the quality of care you so passionately desire to give. So do not lose faith and do not give up hope. It is my prayer that you discover an amazing person buried in the depth of the darkness of dementia. Love will become a dominant element that will shape and protect the relationship.

There is a war going on, but when it comes to dementia, we become confused to what or whom the enemy may be. Some can tend to get mad at the disease or even the person who has it. Many of us fail to see that this disease re-wires the brain. With this change comes a shift in connection points and expressions of love. You will find that you have to become creative in developing a new love language. But the worst thing to do is take a hard-core tactic of going after the disease and the elements that surface within the loved one. There should be a battle, but the battle should mostly focus on fighting to learn and master your new love language and new communication patterns. The battle to know the various elements of where this disease will go and fight to learn the strategies on how to best work within each stage. Follow the signs for how to transition to the next plateau of higher care.

When I use the word "success," there are various ways of looking at what that means. If you have picked up this book and have gotten your interest piqued, the success I am going after is you, as a caregiver, taking pride in the steps you have made to function in that role. Success is being equipped with sound knowledge and techniques to understand the disease and how to respond to what it will throw at you. Success is you creating healthy boundaries and protecting your mental and physical health. Success is you never going it alone. Success is setting up an atmosphere where you can have a connection and deep expression of love to the person you care for while preserving their dignity. Knowledge is power and knowing is half the battle. I want to let you know that I am here for you and will walk you through the other half of winning the battle with great actionable steps. Hang in there and stay confident.

As you witness your loved one's transition, you will see certain skills diminish and the natural response is to rush in and take care of their need. However, with dementia, that can add fuel to the fire and make matters worse because it can make the person feel unpowered. So, from this point forward, I want you to create a new word association when it comes to being a caregiver. I want you to add the phrase "care-partnering" to your vocabulary. What this implies is that you are assisting and guiding them along the corridors of their mind, and you have become so keenly attuned to where this disease will go, that your heroic act of care will assist, shield, protect, and honor who they were while they deal with who they are.

Finding some success
"To do more for the world than the world does for you—that is success." – Henry Ford

Life and time are precious commodities. Once you spend them, you do not get them back. You can invest them, but you do not get an equal or greater return. However, you can manage them. A wise person who controls their life and time will get the best out of every moment. They will cherish these very precious gifts. As we mature, we develop a shifting definition of life. We get to see how fragile it is. We get to understand the importance of giving a high accountability to our life, especially when we engage in caring for the lives of others. When it comes to a person with dementia, it can seem at times like dealing with an unruly child. However, it is actually worse. The wayward child can develop and grow out of it when a dementia patient will only get worse.

In spite of all that I have experienced after being thrust into the depth of care, I feel very blessed and fortunate to do all that I have done. I feel at peace, and I feel empowered. I have come to terms with where this disease leads, but I do not approach it as a loss. I look at it as a release and transition. I realized that much of my stress was coming from my pride and desire. I looked at accepting what this disease will do as a form of giving up, but I now see that I did not give up, I adjusted the rules so that I can win in the area of a blessed relationship. When I began writing this book, my sister was at the stage where she did not remember who I was anymore. I initially felt sorry about it, but there is something magical that emerged from my interaction. We no longer could connect from a point of memory or history, but we could connect at a heart level. She lost her ability to speak, but she could communicate via facial and body expression. I saw her every day at the nursing home. One of the chores that I did for her daily was feed her. She could not feed herself, so she had to be fed. She refused to eat for anyone except me. I believe that the connection we had forged together throughout our years growing up granted the means for me to give her better care.

When I found out that my sister had dementia, I did a lot of research on any known cures. My research led to many dead ends. I contacted many agencies with hope that they would have definite answers. My findings were heartbreaking. My vision looked very dim. I could not just sit back and let my sister suffer through where this disease would take her. As I studied the development of my sister's mind, I had to learn about what my mind was going through as well. I had a fear that this disease could be hereditary as well as being brought on by stress. I had to look at my family history to see if I had other family members who suffered from this disease. I had only detected one other relative with it. That was confirmation for me to take the best in care for myself, to stay aware of the signs, and to improve my personal health. I could not let this disease take anything else from my family. I also had to make some provisions so that my loved ones would have means to love, thrive, and survive with explicit instructions in the event I am ever hit by this disease. I also had to design my life so that stress could not take up permanent residence in my life and home. I had to change my focus and my circle of influences. I had to engage deliberately in things that fuel my spirit and remove things and practices that drain on my spirit and flesh. I had to treat my entire being with an attitude of healthy and sound practices.

I got the glorious privilege to not only do things for my sister but to do things with her. I got to experience her sweet expressions along with a painful emotional expression that this disease frequently produces. I got the opportunity to aid my sister with peace and reassurance when her moments of chaos overtook her. I got a chance to cook for her. She seemed to like much of the foods that I would prepare for her. Above all, through every phase of the disease, I pushed to preserve her dignity.

In contrast, I know it is strange to say, but I love to love myself. Life can condition us to detach and lose site of the fact that our feelings and emotions matter. Society will sometimes persuade you to push your own feelings aside. I had to acquire some valuable skills that enabled me to care and love at the maximum level and to include myself in that equation. When caring for a loved one, especially if that person is your spouse, you can become disheartened and hopeless. I had to get real with the flow of life and know my limitations. I had to learn to let go of the past and to not worry so much about the future that I neglect what I am doing right now. I learned to shape the future that will come. For me, faith played a huge part in my growth process. I was encouraged to value people more, no matter what stage of life they may be in. That enabled me to appreciate the life that I have and examine my contribution I get to make to improve the quality of this world.

Once I broke free from the guilt, pain, and frustration, I was then enabled to care at a higher level of quality. I no longer looked at my sister with resentment but looked at my opportunity to be with her as a gift from God. I was granted the chance to show care in the form of a gift that could not be wasted or returned. I got to look into my sister's eyes and instill a sense of comfort and peace. In her later days, I got to partner with a few nursing homes and hospital staff worker to ensure the quality of her health and the preservation of her dignity. In a way, it has been an enormous blessing for me, because I had much more peace when I interacted with her. I knew that my sister and I would have to say a final goodbye, but God gave us grace and time to be together and to walk in an attitude of peace, freedom, and forgiveness.

I feel much better about myself these days because I do not walk around with a shadow of guilt hanging over me. I feel more empowered about the decisions I make, and I feel empowered to expand my circle of influence when it comes to care. I get to make liberating decisions about the treatment, based not on the stages that are presented to me, but I also base them in conjunction with how I care for myself. This book is not promoting placing your loved in a nursing home but is mainly about the caregivers choosing to put a higher mindset on caring for themselves in order for them to have the level of capacity to care and love for the one under their charge. I can say it has been over a year that I took a vacation day or a holiday because of the intensity of care I was providing. I am sure many of you have gone longer without a break or a day off. Understandably, my sister needed attention, but it is equally wrong for me to totally neglect the fact that I needed to recharge my mental battery.

In February 2015, I was granted the gift of becoming a grandfather for the first time. Once I saw that baby girl, my heart melted. My tough exterior was torn down. When I held her, my spirits were lifted. I felt a rushing flow of life course its way through me. I felt blessed and alive. I made a commitment to be active and healthy. I wanted to be around to spoil her with everything I had. That little princess had me wrapped around her fingers. Her birth also adjusted my priorities of how I was going to treat everything in my life. Balance has to be a staple in my conduct. Additionally, I can say that my experience with learning how to feed my sister has granted me some excellent skills at feeding my granddaughter.

❖Chapter 2 – Help in the Time of Trouble❖

I want to thank you once again for taking this journey with me and for allowing me to share with you. I hope as you read my story you feel blessed, encouraged, liberated, and inspired. I hope you get a renewed sense of hope and a broader outlook of what is ahead and how you can best address it. I can say that my capacity to love has been expanded by how I have chosen to adjust my heart over the quality of care I gave my sister.

Chapter 3 – The Big Picture

"There are many people who can do big things, but there are very few people who will do the small things." – Mother Teresa

All right. Now we are ready to get into the meat of this. Some things will be so simple and obvious, and other things will be eye opening. I am going to walk you through my world of failure and success. There will be so much to learn from both. I will also bring you stories of others that I had the pleasure of encountering along my journey. And at the end of this journey, I hope you can allow your heart to feel elevated and your spirit to be encouraged. There is deep involvement with what you are doing and facing, and I want you to see your value as you do your daily labor of love.

We will be covering the following in detail:

Early warning signs

Many of us who find ourselves in this caring process feel blindsided by the disease. What I want to give you are some practical steps on how to identify if something is a little off and how to know if it is dementia or something else. In this section I also stress the importance of knowing your family's medical history, and I include a few preventative measures that you can take to slow memory loss.

How to get them to get help

Denial is a common response for someone with dementia. However, the way in which we as caregivers approach getting help can drastically affect the health of both your loved one and yourself. One word I want us to add in our vocabulary is "partnering." You want to approach this entire process from a point of view of coming alongside and assisting with a high level of respect. If you can convince them that you are there to protect their interests early on, it will reduce the stress that the both of you may have to experience.

What to expect

I am going to present to you some of the transitional phases I experienced in my sister's journey along with stories of others. I want to help you identify where your loved one is along the scale and equip you with the techniques to ease them into the next progressive level. I will walk you through some effective ways of reacting that will alleviate stress and strengthen the relationship. This section will give you a better idea of what to expect. Your loved one will go through changes that will impact their mind, body and spirit. Lack of preparedness can be a major hindrance.

Early response and lifestyle adjustment

Once you get involved in the care process, there are some changes that could easily become overwhelming. But do not lose hope. When we get to this section, I will talk about the wealth of resources that are out there and direct you on how to construct your support team. You will need this more than anything else when it comes to a healthy care partnership.

Support resources

In this section, we are going to get some very important resources you will need to physically, financially, and medically support yourself and your loved one.

Dealing with legal matters

This section is extremely important. If not handled correctly, you could be limited when it comes to managing assets and making legal decisions. There are going to be some major legal obstacles you will need to face in regard to your loved one's last days especially.

Lifestyle dynamics

This section will implore you to have a healthy pattern of support by giving you a strategy to respond to your loved one's situation with liberty, power, and a shared sense of purpose.

Time Management

This was one of the biggest things that I struggled with, and I had to do a lot of growing to create an environment of health for both my sister and myself. We will explore the dynamics of time and how a person with dementia processes it.

Communications

It does not matter if a person has dementia or is seemingly normal, everyone struggles with communication issues. However, there are techniques you can use to defuse tense situations, and it will create a means to connect heart-to-heart with the one you love. Additionally, there will be some transitions that will take place that impact how your loved one will handle their hygiene, and their activity will greatly impact your overall family dynamics and social life. Handling this will be a powerful transition, but once mastered can create an atmosphere of comfort and trust. It will help you connect in and way with them that makes them feel valued.

Behavior modification

It would be natural to want the person with dementia to behave like they did before the disease, but there will be times when things get rough. There are some simple adjustments you can make that can help them feel confident and assured that they will be safe and comfortable, and that their feelings do matter. There is a powerful force that exists within a thriving relationship. As we look at this section, I want you to look at techniques and tools that will enable you with the skills to get the best out of what you have. There will be some activities you will want to participate in that will help you understand yourself as well as your loved one. This exercise will create a sense of stability for them and a tool that will give you a point of reference steady your relationship with them.

Stress Management

This section is purely for the caregivers. I want to refresh you and help recharge your batteries. You must never neglect yourself. You may come off strong and as a trooper, but the truth of the matter is you are vulnerable, and your tender spot will get hit when you least expect it. This section will give you some tools on how to re-center yourself.

Boundaries and limitations

This section is a short one, but it will talk about identifying what safe and respectful boundaries are and how to transition the boundaries to promote and maintain a safe environment.

Assisted living and nursing homes

Assisted living and nursing homes are a big issue for many with which I have talked. By and large, the disease came as a shock. The impact of the disease gets to be so overwhelming that a decision has to be made to get some major help. However, some of you have already made the commitment never to put them into a nursing home. What to do? I want to walk you through my thought process and see if it can help you identify how you can better care for your loved one with the assistance of trained professionals.

The Long Goodbye

This section is a heavy one for me to address. When I wrote this, my sister had already been in hospice care for three weeks. I watched her health deteriorate every day. Only through prayer was my spirit is at peace for what we faced. I am a person of faith, and it has been my mainstay and what keeps me grounded in the realities that I face while keeping a level head. By no means am I a preacher, or an expert on the Bible or faith, but in this little section, I wanted to impart to you some valuable tools that I have used that transformed my relationship with my sister and that helped me to eventually say goodbye.

Here is the solution

"Impossible only means that you haven't found the solution yet." Anonymous

    I encourage you to set your expectation high. I am going to pour out my best and equip you with some great tools. I am going to guide you through the dark and real world of dementia, and then I am going to flip the lights on. With your eyes opened you will clearly see that you are not helpless. You are not alone. You are not defeated. This is not the end, but it is the beginning of something that has the potential to be beautiful and amazing if you are observant.

    I hope you find this to be a breath of fresh air and totally refreshing to your spirit. This book will change you in some area. It will push you to grow. For me, the things I learned helped me to gain a new perspective on life and what is important. This book will speak to your passion and drive as a human. Please touch base with me online. If you have questions, please send them. I want you to know that we have a community of supporters that will help you walk through all of this.

    We will go over the stages that I witnessed and within some the stages I will go over what I did and outlined if it was right or wrong based on the outcome. At the end of each section, I will outline a list of suggestions on how to best manage the situation with the goal of building a healthy partnership that allows caregivers to show love for themselves as well as for their loved ones without guilt.

Obstacles and objections

"When obstacles arise, you change your direction to reach your goal, you do not change your decision to get there." – Zig Ziglar

Before I jump into the steps and solution, let me talk a bit about some of the things I experienced that limited me. First of all, I felt wounded and blamed God for what I was facing. I was raising a family of my own and just really did not have the time to take care of anyone else. Dealing with this care severely damaged my finances, and I was even unemployed for nine long months. Family and friends that I expected to help slowly drifted away. It also hurt to watch the transition my sister had to go through. It hurt to hear the cutting remarks my sister made which were brought on by the disease. Initially I let these events limit what I thought I could accomplish.

How you overcome obstacles

"When you believe in your purpose you can work through obstacles, and endure hardship." – Bill Cox

First of all, I am so grateful to Jackie Smiertka of the Quality of Life Center in Auburn Hills Michigan. She was my first real resource of help. She loved my sister and provided me assistance, guidance, and coaching. Additionally, the more I talked to others about what I was experiencing, the more I found that I was not in this alone. There are many stories like my own. As we compared notes, we also shared winning ideas that helped the others increase their level of competence to fight this disease. I am also so glad to have friends that were strong in their faith who spoke to me and encouraged me to see the bigger picture of what was taking place with the care I was giving to my sister.

❖ Chapter 3 – The Big Picture ❖

Chapter 4 - Early Warning Signs
"Worry ends when faith begins." – Unknown
What are the early signs?

For many of us, this part is going to feel like jumping into the deep end of the ocean. In general, the early stages of dementia are hard to detect. The subtle changes happen over time and, in some cases, the disease shows itself in behavior. You will find a person, who is usually calm, will start to become more distraught. They will lose track of time; they will develop a pause to their speech pattern as if they are searching for words. As we take a deep dive look into this, I will point out my experience and highlight some other things that I have witnessed in other families I interviewed for my research.

Memory is a treasure. It is only when it begins to slip away that you can truly appreciate its value. When dementia strikes someone, he or she can no longer look at the face of their loved one in the same way, for slowly but surely, that face will drift away. The sands of time carry away the essence of your loved one. The conversations you used to have slowly begin to lose their foundation. Frankly, it is painful to watch someone lose their memories. A spirit of brokenness sets in because a relationship you treasured is, in a way, being slowly stripped away from you. As a caregiver, the advantage you will have by going through this book is having the right frame of mind to know what to expect, and if you know, then you can know what to say and what to do to best aid your loved one. It is largely believed that once the memory cells shut down, they do not come back. But, that does not diminish the fact that you can still be at peace and develop and healthy relationship with your loved one and preserve their dignity and most importantly, protect your personal health.

A pattern of talking about old and not of anything new

This is an interesting pattern to look for and can be quite deceptive when it comes to diagnosing. At times, it will seem as if you are talking to a person who just likes telling old stories, or to a person who is not doing anything new or relevant in their lives. You will find that they will start to tell the story over and over again, or they will tell you the story as if it was the first time they are telling the story. If you find this happening on a regular basis, you should use this a means to increase your curiosity in other areas.

Now, it would be good and respectful to listen to the story and record what they say. The reason for recording their story is that it will help preserve what they have left of their memories. You will find this valuable when you want to share back with them some of their stories. It will show them that their words matter and were valuable enough for you to capture and maintain. You will find that the more respect you can shower them with, the better response you can get out of your loved one. It will also reduce the amount of medication you will have to use to maintain a stable environment.

A classic sign of this disease is that much of the short-term memory will go. They will forget or misinterpret recent things you just said. They will forget scheduled events that they have to attend or appointments to keep. They will forget directions. They will forget people they just met. Things that they have done with routine or people they have known for a long while will become their foundation because they are easier to remember. However, the disease's reach is deep. It will hunt down and pursue every ounce of memory they have and take it from them at will. It is of utmost important that the loss of short term memory is monitored as this is one on the most obvious symptoms of dementia.

Difficulty doing familiar, but difficult tasks – managing money, taking medication, and driving

My sister held a job in which she had to administer vaccines for small children and manage schedules for her clients. Over time, she could not keep up with her appointments, and she began to display much confusion about how to do here day-to-day tasks. Also, she lost track of what to look for when paying her bills on time because in her mind, she was paying all of her bills on time. However, when I reviewed her records and paperwork, I would find checks that were written but never mailed. She also developed a paranoia that people were stealing from her, so she would take and hide and hoard much of her possessions. She would empty out her bank accounts and hide her money under her mattress. This transaction would occur on accounts that she had automatic payments set up on for her bill payments, which would then cause an overdraft on many of here accounts. When we get to the legal section, I will talk about my strategy on how I addressed the money issue.

When my sister was first diagnosed, it was initiated by her supervisor, who was concerned about her work performance and demanded that she be checked out before being allowed to return to work. She went to the doctors and after a few exams, it was determined that she had early, onset dementia. My sister was shocked by what she was told, and her reaction was pure denial. She grew angry and bitter and withdrawn. She hid from family and friends and tried to manage all of her affairs on her own. She was issued medication to help address some of the effects of the disease. However, because of the denial, she refused to take her medication. This had gone on for about six months. Within that short period, she almost lost her home to foreclosure because she forgot to pay her mortgage.

Because she kept her diagnosis secret, and because felt embarrassed about what she was going through, she tried to manage everything on her own. However, she was losing more and more of her cognitive skills and abilities. She would get in her car and travel all over, and there were times when she would get lost and then would struggle to get back home. Her vision was eroding because of the disease, and this was impacting her ability to handle a car safely. So, it got to a point where we had to take her car away from her. This was heartbreaking for her but was extremely necessary for the safety of her as well as the safety of others.

Hindsight has taught me that it would have been good to work with the local authorities about removing her car. It took a while to get my sister to stop driving, but it boiled down to forcing the situation. Consequently, she began to hate those of us who were making a decision to care for her. But, if the mandate came from someone in authority, she would have been more willing to accept it without attacking her caregivers. It is always better to have anger issues displaced onto those in authority. That way, it will reduce any roadblock or resistance you will get while giving care.

Problems with word finding, misnaming or misunderstanding

This is something that everyone struggles with, based on various reasons, but a person with dementia will have more difficulty expressing their thoughts, especially with words or terms that they just learned. They will forget common words, as well as names of people they just met. When they speak to you, they will call you many names that are not yours. The left hemisphere of the brain is one of the first sections of the brain that starts to go. This is your language center. After a time, you will find a person—who used to be talkative—will reduce the amount of what they say. For fear of being embarrassed, they will start to withdraw. Plus, they are losing confidence in what they are saying or feel broken for their loss of words.

Faulty judgement

Hand-eye coordination will gradually fade. You will notice this more when it comes to people who performed a task that required intricate detail. You will see this in people who performed specialized tasks, such as a person who is a surgeon, or a computer programmer, or a person who performs mechanical skills. They will, over time, lose their ability to understand their job, and they will become extremely frustrated and cast blame on others for any shortcoming. They will feel embarrassed about the mistake to the point of doing all sorts of things to cover up their mistake.

It is a good idea for a person with dementia to not make a decision related to any business transient. They should not do any banking or deal with telemarketers. I highly recommend that you set-up conservatorship to protect their checking account from any bad decisions that they may make with their money.

Difficulty problem-solving

The way the human mind works is it takes information and uses it as building blocks for later material, or as a linear string of information. Each brick of information rests upon the next, and information is passed from one connection point to the next. However, when dementia goes to work on a brain, it erodes sections of the brain and the network that distributes information. To solve problems, a person needs a collective functioning brain to possess the skills to solve the problem. With the deterioration of brain cells, it will become harder to solve complex, and at some point, it will even become difficult to solve simple problems. People dealing with dementia will struggle to find words and thoughts, and their brains will send signals that will misdirect them so they will eventually lose the natural systematic means to solve even the basic of life problems.

Misplacing things and putting them odd places

My sister, at the height of the disease, was a master at relocating items. She would wonder the house picking things up that interested her. She lost the ability to differentiate between what belonged to her and what belonged to other people. She had a constant paranoia that people were stealing from her, so she would take everything that she cherished and would hide it all over the house. I found all sorts of mail hidden in odd places that were of a legal nature that never got addressed. You can imagine the headaches that caused. She would even hide food. One day, I went into her room and detected a weird smell. After careful investigation, I discovered that she had hidden food under her mattress, and it had begun to rot. The natural skills that the average person possesses—that allows us to store information—is one of the first abilities that will diminish. Since they have no short term memory, people with dementia will misplace things all the time and in many cases, they will blame the nearest person available for the missing item.

Change in mood or behavior

A person with dementia will have a high level of insecurity. The world that they once knew is slowly being stripped away from them. It is hard to come to grips with what this disease is doing. They are experiencing a constant attack on their brain. When it comes to people helping them out, many feel threatened because they want to feel useful and viable to their environment, and many will fight not to be a burden. Stress levels will run very high, and in some cases, it may not take much to set them off. It is not the case all the time, but this is a classic sign that something is going on with your loved one.

Change in personality

Each day is a new norm for someone living with dementia. The brain is rewiring itself to try to survive. Their personality will change to cope with the internal changes. They will fight to hang on to what once made them feel safe, sane, and stable. A person who leads a highly charged and orderly life, may become a more relaxed and carefree person because the things that used to drive them does not matter to them as much anymore. For others, they may become more threatened by the changes and become resistant, combative or even withdrawn. For still others, I have seen them function with a high level of inhibition and express themselves with crude and vulgar jokes, which they would have never thought of using before the disease.

Loss of interest and withdraw from normal patterns of activities and interest

It is not uncommon for people with dementia to become depressed when they discover they cannot be who they once were. As a result, to cope, many withdraw from people, places and things that they once held interest in. They will seek out a simpler lifestyle or more simple hobbies than they use to do, to just get through their day. Many will spend hours in front of the TV because it is simple, mindless entertainment. Some will change their speech pattern because they have experienced a high loss of words. So, some will choose not speak at all, in order to not embarrass themselves.

Unwarranted bad mouthing

A person with dementia will develop what may seem to be a foul mouth. They will use profanity, racial slurs, and sexual expressions more often. The reason for this is that the area of the brain that acts as a reasoning filter that lets them to know certain words and phrases are taboo is one of the first areas to erode. So there is nothing to stop the barrage of cussing that will take place. However, there are a few techniques you can use to help it become less frequent.

First you must watch for their pattern. There is usually a commonality in the things that trigger the bulk of their foul expressions. In many cases, it will arrive because they are experiencing an extreme amount of frustration. Most people, when they feel stress, whether they have a healthy brain or not, will at least think of a foul word that describes how they feel. In a healthy brain, your modesty center works to prevent you from making socially unacceptable statements. With dementia, there are no barriers, so what is thought off, is expressed. But at the root, it is triggered by some form of frustrating stress.

Mixing up factual events

A person with dementia is still a person. In their mind, they think they are healthy and that the rest of the world has gone bonkers. They are functioning with a less than healthy brain. The methodology used to reason and deduce situations based on the facts that are presented, is a feature that a person with dementia is lacking.

My sister would regularly accuse people of stealing from here. In reality, she would misplace things. However, the brain is extremely logical and demands an explanation for events and behaviors. If something is not where they thought it would be, then the brain will fill in the blank with anything that could make logical sense. Usually, the person who is nearest is the person that gets blamed for taking their things. This is the summary in their mind, and even if they never express their mistrust and frustration in you, it will come across in their interaction with you, and they may be harboring anger over the matter.

You will also find that when they tell a story that they told before, some of the facts and detail of the story will change, simply because the section of the brain that held that fact has either lost the cell, or the neuro-net that carries the information has deteriorated. So the brain fills in the gap of the story with fabricated events either pulled from other memories or other events they may have heard happened to other people. So it pays to be an attentive listener to people in your life. Watch for story details to change and use the previous story as a baseline to determine if your loved one is having a medical issue.

Making 911 calls

This is not as frequent, but it does happen in families and in situations where a person with dementia is not under some form of managed care. The number 911 is very simple and easy to remember. For many of us, it is engraved in our long and short term memory. Those with dementia will have a sense of everything being right and wrong at the same time. There are cases when they get confused, and are desperate enough to ask for help, that they will call 911 for some of the basic things. I have heard of cases of dementia patients who are left alone for a period of time who have called 911 to ask for help with basic instructions, such as how to cook certain food items. They cannot always comprehend that it is an emergency number, and not just a number to call when they need help. You can reasonably believe that something is wrong if your loved is calling 911 on a regular basis for non-emergency matters.

Mixing days and nights

Our bodies have a natural chronometer that helps us sense and keep track of time and events in our lives. As time goes on, you will find that a person with this disease will lose track of time easy. They will forget what day of the week it is, and they will even lose track of what year it is. That is why, in an initial examination, a doctor will ask them if they remember what year it is and what day of the week they think it may be. Trouble equating what day it is is an obvious indicator that there are issues with their cognitive skills.

Shadowing

Because of a loss of certainty brought on by this disease, a person can feel very scared and not quite able to verbalize that they are scared or what causes them fear. So you will find that a person who was once independent will shift to becoming clingier in their body language and mannerisms. They will have a hard time being alone. When they are with you, they will have a higher tendency to touch you, and if you get up and leave their presence, they will be hot on your heels to maintain their level of security. Imagine an infant who, when their parent goes outside of their visual range, will crawl or walk until they see their parent again.

Depression

There are many people in this world who deal with depression. The symptoms of depression can be the feeling of being hopeless, withdrawn, and emotionally shutdown, which can also lead to physical manifestations. It is very easy to get the symptoms of depression mixed up with the symptoms of dementia. If you have loved ones in your life who have become withdrawn, or are talking as though they are losing hold of their life, or are functioning with a broken spirit, you should consider getting them treated by a clinical psychologist. Remember to bear in mind that the same symptoms of depression apply to dementia.

Wandering

Wandering is a big problem that plagues many ambulatory type dementia patients. You will find that wanderers are individuals who are free spirited, quite healthy, have a strong desire to stay physically active, and just want to get out and walk and experience life. However, a person with dementia will have a tendency to walk to far destinations because they still remember how to get there. As dementia sets in, you will find that they will tend to lose their sense of direction, and they will become confused about where they were or where they were going. Since they cannot keep track of time, they cannot tell you how long they have been walking. There are reported cases of some dementia patients who have walked 20 miles or more without knowing how far they have gone away from home. When questioned about their jaunt, they will have no answer as to how far they walked or why they walked. There will be no reason for their walking at times.

I can recall the time during a winter blizzard snow storm that my sister got angry and agitated. Before any of us knew it, she had left the house and began wandering the streets. The difficult part was it was nighttime and the snowfall was blinding. The temperature was around 30°F. I drove down many streets looking at locations where my sister frequented. After driving around for two and a half hours, I just so happened to walk into a store and ask the clerk if they had she seen a woman matching the description of my sister. The clerk had not seen her, and I was getting very discouraged and worried about where my sister could be. I got back in my car and, on the horizon, I noticed a dark figure walking toward my direction. Lo and behold it was my sister. Without a care in the world, she just began walking past me. I was able to get her attention and then got her to get in the car with me. I questioned her about why she left and where she was trying to walk to, but she had no clue that anything was wrong, and she just felt the urge to walk. I quickly dropped the subject because it was evident that it fruitless to discuss it with her. After that incident, we were able to set up safeguards to prevent my sister from leaving the house unassisted.

Rummaging or getting into things

After getting into the deepest realms of my sister's life, I came to the conclusion that my sister had become a hoarder. She picked up anything and everything that she could identify with or that could give her a sense of security. When you feel like you are losing your mind, a common response is to hang on to anything that represents the past and your old passions.

My sister would lay claim to any object that she could get her hands on. Also, one of the side effects of dementia is the modification of one's sensory perception; their fingers become their strong source of stimulus input. People with dementia will touch, pick up, and hold anything that piques their interest. If the object is small enough they will take that object and hide it for a sense of security.

Threatening caregivers

There have been many reported cases of dementia patients verbally and physically attacking caregivers. What many have failed to understand is that many of the attacks are a response to stress and them feeling pressured. There are many things that can trigger a pressured response. It takes a lot of work and understanding on the part of a caregiver to be able to see the signs of stress levels when they are running high. As the symptoms begin to progress, people with dementia will become limited in the variety of responses that they can give. They will be reduced, in some cases, to near animal-like instinct responses. What I had to learn when it came to my sister is that as her brain deteriorated, I had to simplify our schedule and our lifestyle. If she felt pushed, she would get angry fast and express herself. If she felt her dignity threatened, she would get angry and lash out and fight for her dignity, as limited as that might be. The bottom line is what I had to learn was to simply slow things down.

Undressing

This was a hard issue for both my sister and myself. I had to incorporate help with dressing and undressing. However, there were still issues related to how my sister would receive the help that she got. If anyone came on too strong and did not ask my sister's permission before touching her clothes, she would get extremely defensive—and at times combative—because she did not understand why would anyone want to take her clothes off of her. Changing someone else is only possible if it is a joint effort.

Being rude

Some people who struggle with dementia, based on their environment and progression, can tend to come off as being rude. Because of the limited knowledge and training, it is hard to understand where the rudeness or rude expressions may begin. On subsequent sections of the book, I will get into more detail and help you identify if your loved one may be experiencing symptoms of dementia. If you have a loved one that was once calm but is now expressing themselves in a harsh or rude manner, this is a point where you need to consider encouraging them to seek out the physical or medical examination. Rudeness is not reason enough to have your loved one get medically checked. If you see the combination of the aforementioned symptoms, you will then need to work strategically with family members, friends, and even your loved one's employer, to encourage them to seek out a sound medical examination.

Feeling 'sick"

Dementia leads to brain confusion. The person with an advanced stage of dementia may become confused about how their body feels. Their brain tells them that they feel pain. When they describe the pain, and upon examination, you will find that there is no cause for the pain that matches their description. Out of respect and understanding, it is still advisable that they seek medical attention to rule out any physical issues that may cause pain or trauma, but keep in mind that the person with dementia may function as a hypochondriac or exaggerate the slightest pain they feel. They may also have pain that will mysteriously travel around their body.

Striking out at others

We all take our personal space very seriously. When invaded we react. You should expect a more heightened reaction from a person with dementia. You will find that everyone protects their personal space but a person with dementia takes it as a threat that is meant to do them harm. If you find a person is becoming physically aggressive and is inflicting pain on another individual for no apparent reason, this may be a clear sign that they are getting advanced stage brain deterioration. There is a portion of the brain that acts as a filter that controls urges and impulses related to violent tendencies. Once the filter is gone, violence is no longer taboo. It just simply becomes the simplest form of response.

Seeing things and people that are not there

The person with dementia may go through a series of visual changes. A person with normal eyesight will begin to lose their peripheral vision. Over time, they will develop binoculars vision, which will only enable them to see things that are directly in front of them. Over time, they will lose focus. With this factored in, things will not be as they appear to the individual. The brain will come up with its own interpretation of what is being seen.

Eco-ellia – saying things over and over again

This particular symptom is almost on the same level as a person who would stutter. You will find that a person with dementia will be at a loss for words so they will attempt to say a word and mangle it, or they will say a word over and over again to think of the next word that they are trying to say. The right side of the brain controls their native speech, which is also the same section of the brain that deteriorates the earliest. Their vocabulary will dramatically decline. They will lose memory of common words, names, places, and dates. It takes a strong and loving caregiver who is attuned to their loved one to be able to detect this and to lovingly and patiently work with their loved one to get them adequate help.

Resisting care

It is embarrassing to forget things you should know. A person with dementia, especially if they are a proud person who never regularly sees a doctor, will become a challenging case when it comes to seeking out the badly needed medical test to determine the level or type of brain disease they may have. A person with dementia requires a detailed examination by a neurologist and will require a PET scan to determine the level of brain damage, and the PET scan should be done at least twice a year to measure the rate of brain deterioration and which region of the brain is being impacted. However, the big issue is getting them to the doctors for the initial review. Ultimately, I have placed this section in here to make you aware that a person with this disease will become resistant to seeking medical help because it means that they have to give in to the reality of the disease.

You do not fix the disease, you fix the situation

One of the biggest mistakes I made early on was trying to follow the doctor's orders to the letter. Dementia is known worldwide. However, many doctors are limited in how they treat the patient as a whole. One of the fist responses of a general practitioner, or even a neurologist, is to administer a barrage of drugs to address symptoms that the patient may be displaying or things that the caregiver has expressed. However, with every pill comes a side effect. I am sure that many of you have seen the commercials that list the name of the fancy and latest medication, which are followed by so many side effects that the pills seem to not be worth taking. As a caregiver, I will strongly advise you to proceed in this are with extreme caution. The approach I am proposing is if you can know and watch the signs of the onset of dementia, and you can develop a strong and healthy response strategy, then you will greatly minimize the type and amount of medication you will need to maintain good health for your loved one. As of today, there is no cure for dementia. So, from this point out, the focus is a combined healthy lifestyle for your loved one, as well as for you, the caregiver.

Part of knowing the early warning signs of dementia is understanding family history and prevention, so before I close this chapter, I want to discuss the possible risk factors.

Family history, risk factors, and prevention
"If we look into each other's hearts and understand the unique challenges each of us face, I think we would treat each other much more gently, with more love, patience, tolerance and care." – Marvin J. Ashton

If you have had a checkup with a doctor recently, then you will know that a good doctor will dig down into the nitty-gritty and ask the good questions about your family history. They will ask you what do you know about your parent's medical history, as well as your grandparents. They will ask you about traits that have appeared more than once within your bloodline. They want to find out if there are common factors in others to determine the possibility of that factor rising in you. A good doctor will then partner with you on developing preventive lifestyle changes for you to use to empower you to stay at your highest possible level. So take some time and talk to your parents. Also, take the time to do the same for your loved one. Talk to as many relatives as you can and pay attention to things that have impacted your generation and the generation that has gone before. You want to arm yourself with as much information as possible. Once you have gathered all the facts, take some time to read up on the various ailments and examine what treatment your family members have used to address it and find out how well the treatment has worked. Weigh the pros and cons. After you have done your homework, set up your full physical and go in and do a good and thorough workup. After meeting with your doctor and getting any results, you can then work on an agreeable plan on how to address anything that may be found. If they found nothing wrong, you can then at least talk about a plan and regiment to keep yourself at your highest level of health.

Eat brain healthy foods
"At first they will ask you why you are doing it, later they will ask how you did it." – Unknown

I wanted to share with you a list of foods that could be of use to you, as well as to your loved one. If you had the means to promote the best of health to simple eating, would you do it? Then be prepared for empowerment to come from this list of foods that could make life worth living:

1. Curry and Turmeric
These are powerful and commonly used spices that are an anti-inflammatory antioxidant. The key ingredient in these spices is curcumin. Curcumin is capable of crossing the blood-brain barrier and promotes neuroprotection for patients suffering with neurological disorders. Curcumin can help with fighting off the destructive beta amyloids in the brain of Alzheimer's patients, as well as break up existing plaques. Curcumin has even been shown to boost memory and stimulate the production of new brain cells, a process known as neurogenesis. If you were going to go with these spices, I would go with turmeric. This one has a higher concentration of curcumin.

2. Celery

Celery is a rich source of luteolin, a plant compound that may calm inflammation in your brain, which is a primary cause of neurodegeneration. Luteolin has a connection with lower rates of age-related memory loss in mice. In addition to celery, peppers and carrots are also good sources of luteolin.

3. Broccoli and Cauliflower

Kids hate it, but if you want a child to perform well in school, get them started on broccoli and cauliflower as early as possible. They are a good source of choline (Vitamin B), which plays a major role in brain development. An expectant mother who takes Vitamin B during pregnancy "super-charge" the brain activity of babies in utero, indicating that it may boost cognitive function and improve learning and memory. The cool thing is that broccoli and cauliflower may even diminish age-related memory decline and your brain's vulnerability to toxins during childhood, as well as conferring protection later in life.

4. Red Meat

Red meat that comes from grass-fed beef has high amounts of vitamin B12. B12 helps improve cognitive function and also prevents the brain from shrinking.

5. Eggs

When we get older, our brains begin to shrink due to something called brain atrophy. We can fight against this natural process by eating eggs. This is because eggs are full of vitamin B12 as well as lecithin. Vitamin B12 helps to fight against brain shrinkage, as seen in Alzheimer's disease. There is a risk of increasing your cholesterol, so it is recommended that you eat no more than two eggs a day.

6. Walnuts

Walnuts, among many other nuts, are a good source of plant-based omega-3 fats, natural phytosterols, and antioxidants, and have been shown to reverse brain aging in older rats. It contains DHA, which boosts brain function and even promotes brain healing.

7. Crab

One serving of crab contains more than your entire daily requirement of phenylalanine, an amino acid that helps make the neurotransmitter dopamine, brain-stimulating adrenaline and noradrenaline and thyroid hormone, and may help fight Parkinson's disease. Crab is also an excellent source of brain-boosting vitamin B12.

8. Garbanzo Beans (Chickpeas)

Garbanzo beans are one of the best food sources of magnesium (aside from kelp and green leafy vegetables). Magnesium citrate benefits brain cell receptors to speed the transmission of messages while also relaxing blood vessels, which allows more blood flow to the brain.

9. Blueberries

The antioxidants and other phytochemicals in blueberries are directly linked to improvements in learning, thinking and memory, along with reductions in neurodegenerative oxidative stress. They are also relatively low in fructose compared to other fruits, making them one of the healthier fruits available.

10. Healthy Fats

Beneficial health-promoting fats that your body—and your brain in particular—need for optimal function. This includes organic butter from raw milk, clarified butter called organic grass fed raw butter, olives, organic virgin olive oil and coconut oil, nuts like pecans and macadamia, free-range eggs, wild Alaskan salmon, and avocado, for example.

11. Oysters

If you're a seafood kind of person, then today just may be your lucky day. Experiments have shown that oysters are great for your brain, no matter your age. Because they are rich in zinc as well as iron, eating this under-the-sea-delight will help keep your mind sharp and increase your ability to recall information easily. Zinc and iron are linked to the brain's ability to stay focused and remember information. A lack of zinc and iron can result in memory lapses, and poor concentration.

12. Whole Grains

If you have ever tried to lose weight, you know just how healthy whole grains are for your body; however, they are also a great food for your brain. Whole wheat, bran, and wheat germ have high contents of folate, as do brown rice, oatmeal, whole-grain bread, barley, and others. All of these foods work to increase blood flow to the brain which means a higher quality and quantity of brain function. Also, these whole grain foods contain a lot of vitamin B6, which is full of thiamine. Thiamine is great for anyone trying to improve their memory. Scientific research has shown that memory loss dramatically increases by the time you reach your late 60's or early 70's. This means you should eat more whole grains as you get older.

13. Tea

Forget your coffee in the morning- try a cup of tea! Freshly brewed green or black tea is extremely beneficial to your brain because it is full of catechins. Have you ever had a day where you just feel drained, tired, and "too lazy" to think? It may be because you lack catechins in your brain. Catechins are great for keeping your mind sharp, fresh, and functioning properly. Not only do they keep your brain working right, but they also allow it to relax and helps fight against mental fatigue. While green tea is much more potent than black tea, both are extremely good for you. Tea is a great thing to drink early in the morning to ensure you are starting your brain off right.

14. Leafy Green Vegetables

Leafy green vegetables such as cabbage, kale, and spinach, while not very well-liked by children, are excellent for the brain of children and adults alike. These vegetables greatly help when it comes time to remember old information and process it like you just learned it yesterday. This is because these foods are often full of vitamin B6, B12, and folate, which are great compounds needed within the brain to break down homocysteine levels, which can lead to forgetfulness and even Alzheimer's disease. These vegetables are often very high in iron content. If there is not enough iron intake, cognitive activity slows down greatly. So when mom always urged you to eat your spinach, now you know why.

15. Fish

Eating fish overall is greatly beneficial to your health, especially that of your brain. Fish is full of Omega-3, which is a fatty acid known to be highly beneficial to the body for various reasons. Eating one serving of fish a week can greatly decrease one's chances of getting Alzheimer's disease. These fatty acids help the brain function because they coat the neurons that at times have a fatty acid layer that becomes stiff due to a high content of cholesterol and saturated fat in the body. Omega-3 will coat the neurons with good fat, allowing them to move easily throughout the brain. Omega-3 also provides more oxygen to the brain, as well as allows one to retain new information while still remembering old information. The best fish to eat for brain health are salmon, tuna, and herring.

16. Chocolate

While eating hundreds of *Hershey's* bars may make you sick, and drinking a lot of hot cocoa in a day just may do the same, the main ingredient in these oh-so-delicious foods, cocoa, is said to be very nutritious for the brain. Scientists have proven that the antioxidant content found in just two or three tablespoons of cocoa powder is much stronger than that found in other foods, such as green tea or red wine. The main antioxidant found in cocoa, known as flavonols, is said to help increase blood flow to the brain. While normal milk chocolate lacks flavonols, you will find plenty of it in dark chocolate.

Challenge to learn

"When were are no longer able to change our situation, we are challenged to change ourselves." – Viktor Frankl

Just as if you wanted to train your body for a major event, such as the iron man race, so you should train your brain for the game of life. You should find non-routine things to do that push you outside of your element. You will find that you will keep your brain in growth mode. If you decline in your learning challenges, you can put your brain in a sedentary state and over time you will lose your capacity not only to learn, but your short term and long term memory may become inhibited.

Music

"Music is the prayer the heart sings." – Unknown

Music has a powerful and deep reach into our soul. Music moves you. Music can be a part of our identities. You can almost define a person's region and culture by the type of music that is in their playlist. I remember that when I was growing up I had difficulty learning in school. However, I had a deep love of music. So I had to learn how to blend music into the harder subjects that I had to learn for it to stick and make sense. School House Rock saved my life.

One area of music therapy could be the practice of listening to music that you do not usually have interest in. For instance, if you are big on listening to country, try listening to jazz, or pop, or even spiritual music. Look for music outside of your realm, and it will have the potential to enhance your brainpower. You can take it a step further by challenging yourself to memorizing the lyrics of some new songs.

New language

"One language sets you in a corridor for life. Two languages open every door along the way." – Franck Smith

My base language is English, however, I have traveled the world and in every country I visited, I had a translator who was available to help me navigate the language for the people with which I needed to communicate. It would have been more liberating if I had taken the time to learn the local language. I would have had a much richer experience. With that said, learning a new language can be challenging, but it is the perfect challenge that your brain needs to stay in learning mode. The longer you keep your brain in learning mode while reducing stress, the healthier and more protected your brain will be. So, get a copy of *Rosetta Stone* and have at it.

Chapter 5 - How to Get Them to Get Help?

"Encouragement is the fuel on which hope runs." – Zig Ziglar

This will probably be a challenging section for some of you to go through. What do you say to your loved one who you see having some difficulties navigating their once simple life? It is painful to watch them struggle, but it can be scary and difficult to persuade them to get help. My experience with my sister was a nightmare. However, hindsight and research have taught me a much better approach. It is not an exact science, but the strategy that I present next will move you close to the mark.

Do not force

It is hard enough for a single person to manage their own life, let alone take on the responsibility of managing someone else's life. What I want to stress here is that the amount of time and energy you put into getting them to get help will be the same level of time and energy you will put into its maintenance. If you have to force them to get help, you will create an uphill battle for yourself. No one wants to be bossed or pushed around, especially when it comes to getting medical attention. This resistance is multiplied because they do not feel that they are sick.

You will want to show sensitivity as you express your concern. They may be confused and scared, so you will need to key in on where they are and gradually move them into a healthy environment where they feel safe and empowered to talk about how they feel and what they think they may be experiencing. Keep in mind that a person who is experiencing the initial stages of this disease may likely feel isolated withdrawn and alone. The world that they know and could solidly stand upon is slowly being eroded right from under them. It is a hard transition they are going to have to make. To force them to get help will make them either respond with a fight or flight attitude. You will want to ease them slowly into an atmosphere of health.

Share your empathy

What acts as a great icebreaker for getting your loved one help is for you to delve into your own personal vulnerability. You will want to come up with a story that talks about how you had to get to the point in your life where you knew you were out of your depth and needed help to address what you were facing. Talk about the reassurance it gave you and about how it made it better for everyone around you. If your loved one can sense your vulnerability, then it will make it easy for them to open up and share what they may be experiencing.

Don't debate—relate through questions

Remember, for this discussion, there is no *right* or *wrong*, and there is no *winner* or *loser*. You want to create an atmosphere where your loved one feels safe to talk to you about how they feel and any symptoms they may be experiencing. You will want to use leading questions that help them to feel safe to express their vulnerability while preserving their dignity. A possible dialogue could begin with the following: "I know it must have been a little frustrating today when you got lost while driving. You have gone that route over a hundred times. Do you think it may be a good idea to talk to your doctor to see if they can give some suggestions on what you can do to help with your memory?"

Whatever you do, do not hammer them about how they *must* see a doctor. You should use a series of subtle questions. Use questions designed to move them to a vantage point where they can better see how advantageous it would be to get a check-up. You want to ask questions in such a way that they feel as if it was their idea to see a doctor and that it is safe to get help and support. Let them know how much you love them and how much you depend on them and that because of what you are witnessing, it is harder for you to feel assured in relying on them. Let them know how it hurts you to watch them go through so much. Let them know that it would just give you some peace of mind to pursue getting a simple checkup.

Find common points of agreement

Before you start the conversation, make a list of issues that you have witnessed that may be of concern to you. Bear in mind, you are not going to function like you are in a courtroom and trying to win a trial. It is stressful to your loved one to try to pin them down on any issues. You will need to take a subtle approach and get them to talk and express themselves. Let us take forgetfulness, for instance. You can get them to talk about how it made them feel to forget certain simple things. You do not want them to feel pressured or embarrassed. Only talk about what they are willing to express. If you press, they will withdraw and feel threatened and alienated by you. You want to create an atmosphere where they feel loved. You will want to reassure them of this many times throughout your conversation.

Here are ten starter questions to see if you can find a point of agreement. Keep in mind that if a person can answer yes to five or more of these issues, it is highly recommended that they seek medical help even if you may not suspect dementia.

1.   How often have you forgotten or missed important dates or events, or find yourself asking for the same information over and over or having trouble remembering people's name or important phone numbers?

2.   Do you ever get frustrated dealing with numbers, or following a recipe when cooking, or have trouble keeping track of your bills, or do you feel you need more time to get things done more than usual?

3.   Do you ever feel you have issues with places you have to drive to or find you are having difficulty controlling your car or do you find it much more difficult to do your job?

4.   Do you ever forget what year, day or season you are in, or do you ever forget where you are or how you got to a certain location at times?

5.   Do you feel that you are having trouble with your vision when it comes to judging distance or colors, especially while driving?

6.   Do you find you have trouble spelling common words, or ever forget words or what they mean, or do you forget the names of people you have known for quite some time?

7.   Have you lost anything as of late, or misplaced something and had trouble finding it?

8.   Have you bought anything from a telemarketer or find that you paid too much for something?

9.   Do you find yourself losing interest in hobbies that you loved to do, or are there social groups or church functions you have stepped away from or have you stopped hanging with family or friends?

10.   Do you ever feel confused, suspicious, depressed, fearful or anxious or do you find yourself easily upset at home, at work, with friends or in places where they are out of your comfort zone?

Start small

To get an accurate diagnosis of dementia or Alzheimer's requires an examination by an experienced neurologist and even a PET scan. However, the sound of those tests seem intimidating and overwhelming. The smarter approach would be to sit down with your loved one and help them to make out a list of their symptoms and then have them take that list to their general practitioner. This will be helpful for building a good foundation for treatment. You can then leverage their doctor to seek out further testing with a neurologist. It will prove to be a good idea, in the long run, to make their doctor and others that are in authority the bad guy when giving heavy news or directions. This will serve to increase your loved one's trust in you.

Partner with them

One issue I wish I could have changed when it comes to my sister's care would have been attending some of her early doctor appointments with her. My sister went a year trying to manage her health on her own. That year cost her dearly when it came to the quality of her life. The efforts we took to correct things were too little too late.

What you want to establish a team-like relationship with your loved one in which they are leading and you are there to assist. You want them to cooperate with you for the simple fact that you want them to sign a HIPPA form that authorizes a doctor to talk to you on their behalf. If not, you will not be given a full picture of what your loved one is facing medically.

Seek higher help

Right out of the gate, you will seek out help from anyone and everyone that could directly or indirectly help you. You will want to talk to the Alzheimer's Association and any other local resources if you need at-home care or are seeking adult day care. You will need to seek out counseling for yourself to make sure you are keeping yourself balanced.

As you talk to other professionals, try to ask for advice that may be of assistance with what you may be going through. There are tons of resources out there, so take advantage of them the right way and as often as possible. I strongly recommend reading the rest of this book and also do a lot of research at ALZ.org. There are a wealth of resources available there that could equip you for success and building or maintaining a healthy relationship with your loved one.

Build your team

There are some caregivers who have taken the lone wolf approach. They have cared so hard, so deep, and with so much passion, that they did not realize how they alienated others in their life and, to a degree, became a martyr. This disease is slow and takes a lot from you as a caregiver. To be effective, you will need to become a better communicator and organizer. If you try to take it all on, you will find that some of your closest loved ones will let you carry the burden, until it breaks your back. So, be wise straight out of the gate, and invite as many family members, friends, church family members, and club affiliations to help out. You will find that as time goes on, your team will drift away. Tell yourself that it is all right and natural. Having this team early on will help you build up other resources to help you prepare for the next phase of the journey.

Lean on love

You will need to connect heart-to-heart with your loved one. You will need to express yourself in a way that helps them to know and feel how bad it is making you feel to see them in the way they are functioning. Be honest and talk from the heart. And with hope, they may choose to seek out help. Above all, do not beg, pressure, demand, or force them to get help. It will just create a world of stress that will make treating the disease very unpleasant and possibly harmful. As a last resort, if your loved one gets to a point of depression where they are becoming combative or are talking about committing suicide, then you will have to go around them to get urgent help. At that point contact their doctor, the local ER or call 911.

Going deeper

Meet with your loved one's doctor and work out a strategy once you get the HIPPA form signed that allows the doctor to talk to you. You will then need to schedule a meeting with the doctor to develop a treatment strategy collectively. You will find this to be very valuable because you will better understand what is going on medically. Additionally, I am going to push that you learn as much as you can about your loved one's medical history and take a good look at the type of drugs prescribed. You will need to know what each drug does and look at the side effects. It is especially important to know how each drug may counteract with other drugs.

Many general practitioners will treat the disease with drugs, but my experience has taught me that this will do more harm than good. When I started dealing with my sister's treatment, she started with three types of medicine and worked her way up to eight different pills a day. Over time, the chemicals built up in her system, but at the same time her body was fighting it, so we had to keep upping the doses. All the drugs, in my opinion eventually caused her to start having seizures.

Just as I am encouraging you to partner with your loved one, I am equally suggesting you to partner with the doctor. All of this may seem like a lot of work, but if you ignore doing this, you will find that a lot more work will generate on the back end of the disease. You will want to utilize every ounce of help and resources that you can to develop a sound response plan. A person with dementia will be a wild card, and you want to build up an adequate list of responses to address what you may experience so you can be proactive and not reactive.

Getting a proper neurological exam and a PET scan

As you move them beyond the general practitioner, and they get the initial exam from and neurologist, you will want to request a Positron Emission Tomography (PET) scan. This is a scan that utilizes radiation or nuclear medicine to produce a 3D mapping of the brain. It will give the doctor a clear map that shows what portions of the brain are functioning. You will want to get this scan done on an annual basis so you can track the progress of the disease. This test can, along with blood and lab work, help narrow down the type of dementia and will help you develop a better treatment plan. By getting this scan done annually, you can rate how fast the disease is progressing and what sections of the brain are deteriorating the fastest. A PET scan will give you a better idea of what to expect from your loved one that will help you with your sound response plan.

Only 2 out of 10 get a good evaluation

Later in this book we will get deeper into the various types of dementia. There are quite a few and each one is treated differently. However, the diagnoses are extremely vital. Practically everyone has heard of the word dementia, but many do not understand what it is and what it can do until faced with it or are caring for someone who has it. When it comes to medical science, the experience and background on this disease has not fully caught up to the medical community. This disease has been around for many years, but the science on it has only been around for the past 15 years. It is growing at an epidemic proportion. There are not enough highly trained doctors that know how to come up with a healthy treatment plan, other than prescribing medication to address symptoms.   Unfortunately, only two out ten patients get a good diagnosis. So the majority of people living with dementia have their disease treated in an incorrect manor.

Test for high levels of Plasma Homocysteine

Even if you have heard of the term "hardening of the arteries," you probably did not know that it is related to the build-up of homocysteine. This is an amino acid that can build up too much protein in your arteries. A simple blood test can reveal if any of protein levels are high. If discovered early enough and treated thoroughly, it could prevent heart issues. This same element is a large contributor to plaque build-up in the brain, which will reduce oxygenated blood supply, which will lead to cell damage and memory loss. Once a brain cell dies, it cannot be repaired.   So it is imperative to keep your blood supply oxygenated through good blood flow and to lead a very active life that includes cardiovascular activity.

MCI – Mild Cognitive Impairment

I feel that a person should be involved with activities that challenge their brain.   The challenges improve your brainpower, but it also acts as a gauge to measure your brain health.   I encourage games that utilize memory skills.   Through regular practice, you will be able to see where you are experiencing memory loss. Memory loss is a natural part of aging. However, the memory loss can be kept at a minimal if we practice a healthy lifestyle.

When it comes to a person that is experiencing dementia, they will have mild cognitive impairment

(MCI). This will be a noticeable memory loss that will occur daily. They will lose the ability to store new information. The short-term memory is the first area of the brain under attack and experiences the plaque buildup that kills off the active brain cells. To detect this development, you will be required to have regular contact with your loved one so you can measure and gauge their activity. I recommend you keep a journal of what you are witnessing and take it with you when you go to see their doctor. It will aid the doctor with how to better treat the symptoms.

Family history

It is not definite that if dementia runs in your family you will get it. However, there is scientific evidence that points to the disease potentially passing down generationally. One common factor is there is high plaque build-up in the brain. If you have a history of high cholesterol, diabetes, heart disease or blood pressure issues, your risk of getting dementia is increased. I would recommend that you encourage every member of your family to get regular check-ups and if you have some high-risk factors, utilize your doctor's help to get them under control. It will at least help you know where you stand with maintaining a healthy lifestyle.

What I'm proposing that you consider, as a member of your bigger family unity, is that it would be a good idea for you to talk to as many family members as you can about getting an annual health screening. There are a lot of things a person could prevent if they had the right information and a working strategy on how to address any possible health issues. If health is a common topic of talk in your family, it makes it a lot easier to talk to any of your loved ones about getting help when they are showing serious signs of things being wrong. Also, if you are encouraging your family unit to seek out good screenings, it makes it easier to develop a good support system if any of your loved ones should happen to experience a debilitating disease.

Overall phases

So, what is dementia? That is a big question and, to many, it is confusing because there are so many types. One of the more common terms that people hear is Alzheimer's. Alzheimer's is a subset of dementia. It is important to know the medical symptoms of dementia in its many forms because you will not only recognize them in yourself and others, but you will be able to give specific examples of what the body is going through when someone has the disease. This knowledge might persuade your loved one to get help. According to the Alzheimer's Association, some of the medically related signs are:

1. Plaques - microscopic clumps of protein fragments, called beta-amyloid.
2. Tangles - microscopic twisted strands of the protein tau (sounds like "WOW!").
3. Disconnect - the neuro-network that ties the brain cells together to transfer information becomes disconnected. These cells control memory, learning, and communication.
4. Inflammation - the brain experiences swelling triggered by the body's immune system.

5. The death of brain cells - on a daily rate, sections of the brain cells that house information ceases to function and brain tissue shrinks.

Some of the common types of dementia are as follows:

Alzheimer's - Most common cases come from this making up an estimated 60 to 80 percent of the reported cases. For a person with Alzheimer's, many of the symptoms will develop and show well before the disease diagnosis. Some of the symptoms include an inability to remember recent conversations, names or events, a loss of interest in activities and events they would normally do, and depression.   As the disease progresses, impaired verbal communication, poor judgment, disorientation, confusion, rapid mood change, and difficulty, walking, talking and swallowing also become factors.

Vascular dementia - This makes up about ten percent of the reported cases. It is brought on as an aftereffect of a stroke. Initially, a person will have an inability to make a decision, plan, or organize. There are not many issues with memory loss, but mostly confusion. This is a result of bleeding related to ruptured blood vessels or vessel blockage. These ruptured or blocked vessels can be discovered via a PET scan. With the advance in technology, the ruptures can be repaired, however, any restricted oxygenated blood flow to sections of the brain, may cause irreversible brain damage.

Dementia with Lewy bodies (DBL) – This disease will match the memory issues of Alzheimer's, but it will also include sleep disorders and visual hallucinations, along with muscle rigidity or other Parkinsonian's movement features. This form of dementia comes from a clumpy build-up of alpha-synuclein protein within the cortex section of the brain just like in Parkinson's disease.

Mixed dementia - This could be a mixture of the symptoms a person would get from Alzheimer's, vascular dementia, or DBL.

Parkinson's disease - This disease attacks the portion of the brain that controls motor skills. It most strongly resembles dementia with Lewy bodies. Alpha-synuclein protein clumps form in a substantial section of the brain that will lead to degeneration of nerve cells that produce dopamine.

Frontotemporal dementia - This is brought on by a microscopic abnormality. It can be caused by frontal head trauma or in some cases, genetics. A person with this disease has fewer years life expectancy than someone living with Alzheimer's. It impacts the personality and behavior, language development, and the front and sides of the brain.

Creutzfeidt-Jakob disease (CJD) - If you have ever heard of "Mad Cow Disease" then you may recall that this is a brain disorder that can transfer between humans and animals. This disease rapidly erodes the memory and the formation of misfiled prion proteins that rapidly spread throughout the brain. It impacts motor skills and coordination, as well as moods and behavior.

Normal pressure hydrocephalus (NPH) - This disease comes from a build-up of fluid in the brain. It will impair walking, memory, and the ability to control urination. This is one of the few controlled types of dementia, and it can sometimes be corrected with a surgical installation of a shunt for draining the excess fluid.

Huntington's disease - This is a genetic defect that impacts chromosome 4. A person with this will experience abnormal involuntary movements, recessed reasoning skills, and a heightened irritability, along with depression and a wide variety of mood swings. It is a slowly progressing disease.

Wernicke-Korsakoff syndrome - This disease is commonly brought on by a high amount of alcohol use. The alcohol build up helps promote a deficiency of thiamine (vitamin B-1). This could impact memory but still allow the person to function socially without too much difficulty. The brain functions off of sugar. The thiamine helps the brain cells produce energy from the sugar. So basically, the brain is not functioning at peak efficiency.

The stages of dementia

If you are dealing with a loved one with dementia, it is vital and empowering for you to know the phases of the disease. With this knowledge you will be well equipped to respond in the healthiest of ways.to their worsening condition. In the medical world, there are five stages of progression for this disease. This addresses some of the commonalities among the different types of the disease. The rating system is better known as the Clinical Dementia Rating (CDR). The five stages describe a patient's ability to perform in six different areas of cognition and functioning: orientation, memory, judgment, home and hobbies, personal care, and community.

Stage 1: CDR-0 or No Impairment

Stage one of the CDR is the baseline of someone with a good sound mental and neurological state. If your loved one gets a score of 0, they have no detectable issues. They show no time displacement, they exercise good judgment, they can interact in a social setting, they can manage their home life, and they are classified to handle financial, medical, and legal affairs.

Stage 2: CDR-0.5 or Questionable Impairment

If your loved one gets a score of 0.5 on the CDR scale, it means they are showing some obvious signs that are suspect and will require some further investigation. What a doctor will be looking for is a person showing a pattern of memory inconsistency, problem-solving, and time displacement. Another obvious sign will be that they are slipping or falling behind at work on a regular basis, or that they may seem to struggle in or withdraw from social situations. This person may not be qualified to work, but they still have enough mental ability to manage their personal care without any help.

Stage 3: CDR-1 or Mild Impairment

At a CDR level 1, they have shifted to showing some obvious signs of impairment in memory, thought processing, motor skills, as well as work and personal tasks and may struggle in a social setting. The short-term memory loss is more obvious and starting to impact their daily routine. They will tend to get lost or turned around very easily. Outside of their element, they will struggle quite a bit. You will notice in the home, daily activities are being neglected such as chores and hygiene.

Stage 4: CDR-2 or Moderate Impairment

Once they move into this stage, your loved one will need help and assistance with practically everything. Sometimes they will need more patient direction and in other cases, they will need to have certain things done for them. They will require a lot of assistance with hygiene. They may have enough awareness about themselves that will enable them to function in social settings and to do chores to a limited degree, but they will have to be monitored at this point. They will be much more confused with time and directions. At this point, there will be a significant impairment of the short-term memory. You will notice this by the frequency of questions you may get from your loved one or they will repeat stories they have told before.

Stage 5: CDR-3 or Severe Impairment

At this stage, things intensify. Your loved one will need direct and around the clock care. They will need help with every stage of anything they are doing.

Many who make it to this stage, will need either full-time care from a series of loved ones, or a visiting nurse. If they are at an intense level, they will need to transition to a nursing environment, based on the level of care they may need and the level of care you will be able to construct for them.

Progressive Dementia

Once again, by being aware, you can then plan ahead on how you want to choose to respond. You can pre-plan for help and support as well as living arrangements and long-term care. For some forms of the disease, you may be able to slow some of the effects by implementing some healthy lifestyle adjustments and improving the quality of life. At the same time, be ready to address the transitions when you start to see the signs of the disease. Please note, there are some forms of dementia that are revisable. If the dementia is caused by an infection, nutritional deficiency, as a side effect of a medication, or from brain bleeding, the symptoms can be stopped and reversed as long as the underlying cause is treated.

Various diseases that may cause misdiagnoses:
Narcissistic Personality Disorder

A person with this disease will act in a way where they want to draw attend to themselves for the purpose of being superior, and this is mostly used as a form of overcompensation to cover up some form of shame or fear they may have experienced. A person displaying these symptoms may not have a memory issue as much as they do a truth issue. Much of this can be addressed through psychotherapy. The misdiagnosis comes into play when a person with this disease fabricates a fable and interprets it as a memory problem.

Antisocial Personality Disorder (ASPD)

A person with this disease does not have a problem with being antisocial, but they do have a problem with respecting the rights, feeling and emotions of others in a social setting. This is a person that has been exposed to an environment lacking any moral common sense. They may have been exposed to people with criminal tendencies or an environment loaded with aggressive behavior. The part where it gets confused with dementia is that people with dementia lose their inhibition, so they tend to use foul language and vulgar expression. So with ASPD, a person is acting a certain way because of social conditioning, whereas with a person with dementia, they are like a loaded gun with the safety broken off. They feel the need to restrict of defend anything they are expressing.

Borderline Personality Disorder (BPD)

This is an extremely impulsive person. They are driven by circumstances, and their responses could be an extremely high or an extremely low and it could change on a dime. They could be happy one moment and become extremely rough and rude the next. What distinguishes this from dementia is signs such as loss of memory, along with the cognitive skills loss.

The confusion with the diagnosis comes in when a person with dementia will display mood swings as a means to compensate for the fear and stress they are under because of the confusion they are experiencing. A person with BPD has more means to control their expression with the help of good psychotherapy, counseling, and behavior modification.

Bipolar Affective Disorder

A person with bipolar disorder will experience mood swings and, in some cases, psychosis and hallucinations. There are some similarities between bipolar and dementia. However, the mood swings with bipolar affective disorder are based on how the brain is firing and being fueled by sugar, whereas the mood swings that a person with dementia commonly display come from a reaction to emotional simulation and their fight to make sense of what they are experiencing because of the loss of memory.

The brain map

Before we move from this section, it is important to understand the different functions of each section of the brain to better understand it yourself and to better explain it to your loved one dealing with dementia. The human brain is made up of three major parts: the cerebrum (memory, emotions, logic and motion), the cerebellum (balance and coordination), and the brain stem (connects to the spinal cord and controls automatic functions of organs such as the heart and lungs). With a single heartbeat, approximately 25% of your body's blood is pumped to your brain. In that blood is oxygen, sugar, and protein. Within that same heartbeat, billions of cells use about 20% of the oxygen housed within your blood. There is a network of veins and capillaries, which is known as the whole vessel network.

When you see a picture of a brain, you see wrinkles all over. This section is called the cortex. Near the very top of your head, in the center, this section controls how your body sensors work. The section of the brain just above the brain stem controls sight. The section of the brain that controls sound is on the right side of the brain, just above the ear. The section that controls how you smell things is on the underside of the brain near the front base. The frontal lobe controls how you think and solve problems and make plans. The section of the brain on the right side near the ear controls how memories are stored. The section on the top of your head, toward the front, controls voluntary movement.

The left brain controls the right side of the body, and the right side of the brain controls the left. For most people, the center of speech is on the left side of the brain.

An adult human brain contains over 100 billion nerve cells called neurons. Each cell has multiple connection points that branch out. An average brain has about 100-trillion connection points. This is your neuron-network or neuron forest. The network is how thought and memories travel through the brain. Neurons are the main section of the brain that gets attacked when someone had dementia. For memory or decision-based thought to travel in the brain, a tiny electrical charge is required. The point where the nerve cell connects is called the synapses. As a charge travels through the synapses, it releases a neurotransmitter. Alzheimer's disrupts the electrical current and the release of the required neurotransmitters.

When Alzheimer's hits, it completely re-wires the brain and how the system functions. Alzheimer's causes nerve cell death and deteriorates tissue mass. This damage impacts the overall function of the brain along with many other body functions.

Over time, the cortex shrivels, especially in the hippocampus area which is vital for storing new memories.   Cavities form—called ventricles—that increase brain fluid that impair memory function.

A person with Alzheimer's or dementia has fewer nerve cells and synapses. Protein plaque forms in between the nerve cells that block the transfer of information. Dead and dying brain cells contain a twisted strand of proteins called tangles. Scientists have not yet concluded what the cause may be for the cell death or tissue loss, but in every case plaques and tangles have been commonly found.

Plaques come from a build-up of a sticky protein called Beta-Amyloid, which is a fragment of a larger protein found in the fatty membrane surrounding the nerve cell. Once you get enough of the Beta-Amyloid to attach, it cuts off the synaptic flow to the nerve cells. It also activates the immune system to attack the living brain cells and to fight it as if it is an infection.

When it comes to the brain and the transfer of information, you can think of it like the Internet. The Internet is modeled after the human brain and neuro-network.   You have computers that are all over the world that are loaded with all sorts of information, some valuable and some trivial.   They are all linked together by a powerful and elaborate network that is fast and redundant and has the power to transfer large amounts of information from point A to point B in a fraction of a second.   When you plug your computer into the network, you are then allowed to tap into the World Wide Web. But perhaps your power goes out or your wires get broken or your router is down. If you are working on something critical, then you are dead in the water. Imagine you were running your business from home and your network went down. For some, a few minutes could mean an eternity.   And for some businesses, if they are down for that long, it could cost the future of the company and may eventually kill the business.

Just like the Internet, you have a network coordinated in a nice and orderly series of strands of information transports in your brain. To sure up the strength of the network, a protein called Tau is present. As dementia is active in a brain, it as if the Tau protein breaks down and starts to twist and the twist causes a short in the brain wiring and causes that network connection to short out and die. That twist is also referred to as tangles. With the lack of flow of nutrients and information, the nerve cell eventually dies.

For a person diagnosed with dementia, their life expectancy and rate of progression is determined by the age it was discovered as well as any other pre-existing medical condition, along with their lifestyle. A person with dementia has a life expectancy of eight to twenty more years after the initial diagnosis. People with early Alzheimer's can have symptoms that come on slow, and gradual changes could take place over a 20-year time span even before they get diagnosed. A person with mild to moderate Alzheimer's have between two and ten more years. Severe Alzheimer's may give a person only about one to five years.

In the initial stages of the brain attack, the central portion of the brain and frontal lobe are broken down. This section of the brain controls a person's ability to learn new things and to maintain short-term memory. The frontal lobe controls the logic and reasoning.

In the mild to moderate stage, the areas that control the memory and thinking will have a considerable amount of plaques and tangles and cell detention. The loved one will have a significant memory loss that will impact their daily activity and work. At this stage, you will need to file for social security disability if that financial need is required. The confusion level will be much higher, and they will have a lot of trouble handling money, speaking, and communicating. Their thoughts will become very confusing, and they will have difficulty making sense of things that will lead to a lot of frustration. Usually, a person will display these changes around the time they are first diagnosed with dementia or Alzheimer's. The next area of the brain that is impacted are the parts that control speech and the ability to interpret speech. They will also lose a sense of where they are and will not recognize the objects that are around them. As it progresses, they will experience changes in personality and begin to lose the identity of loved ones around them.

Once they advance to the severe stage, they lose a great deal of their cortex and brain stem due to the death of many cells. They will lose their ability to communicate, to recognize family, and to control bodily functions.

Chapter 6 – What to Expect (Changes You Will See over Time)

"When you stop expecting people to be perfect, you can like then for who they are." – Donald Miller

Since I have already walked you through some of the scientific changes a person can go through with dementia, I will now walk you through some of the things I experienced with my sister that you might not otherwise understand from medical resources.

Sleep management

When my sister was well, she was an active person. She stayed busy and active and on the go. She hated sitting still. She had a love for travel and meeting people and doing new things. However, I noticed some changes in her behavior as the disease began in its initial stage.

My sister's sleep schedule became very irregular. When she was working, she would set her alarm to a loud level. When the alarm would go off, it stayed loud and steady for an hour before she would hear and respond to it. At first, I thought her ears were going bad, but when she was awake, she heard things perfectly fine. However, her internal clock was deteriorating, and she was developing a lack of response to certain sounds, almost on the same level of selective hearing.

Over time, after being placed on sick-leave from work, she would then take random naps throughout the day. This in turn caused her to stay up all night watching TV or wandering around the house. I eventually got her started on a sleep aid to help her rest at night, which was a strong narcotic and the side effect impacted her mental state. I would recommend a milder sleep aid, called *Melatonin*. It is over the counter, and it does not leave any nasty after effect in the system, and it allow the person to get peaceful sleep.

As a caregiver, because of my sister's lack of rest, it made it considerably hard to work with her in the day or the night, and it impacted her mood. It created a lot of stress when interacting with her. It is important that you gently persuade them to get on a sleep schedule that is in sync with your own. If you are not getting good rest, then you will put your personal health at risk and will can eventually render you incapable of providing care for your loved one as well as other areas of your life.

Roll change adjustment

This was a hot issue for my sister. My sister was 12 years older than me and had a Type A personality. She was a leader and vocal, and she was not the type to bend to authority. She was in denial of the disease for a long time before she would allow herself to get help. There was a considerable amount of damage done to her brain by the time she allowed anyone to step in to assist.

My sister had a hard time transitioning from being a leader to being assisted. She hated the fact that her daughter and her younger brother had to take some form of authority over her life and decisions, along with her day-to-day activities. She hated that someone was managing her schedule.

The disease hits and overwhelms many with a flood of emotions that they do not have the full mental capacity to control or comprehend what they are feeling. So, to relate, I had to learn to adjust the framework that was healthy for both of us to operate within. I had to create a false premise to make her think that she was always in charge while planting suggestions for what I needed her to do. I had to learn that I could not come at her strong, and I had to respect her natural boundaries. I had to get in the practice of asking her permission or her advice on things to get her opinion before offering a suggestion on anything that I needed her to do. I had to adjust the conversation to make it seem like the thing that I wanted her to do was her own idea. Once she felt that she granted permission, she then was more agreeable to do whatever needed to get done. I will get into more detail of what that looks like later in the book.

Awareness of a new center of balance and gravity

As my sister got about half way through her stages with the disease, I noticed that she was walking bent over. I thought she was hurt or something, so at times I would try to assist her and make her stand or sit up straight, and seconds later, I would find her bent over again. What I later found is that because she had Lewy Bodies Dementia, one of the side effects was the hardening of the muscles. It is as if someone had turned on that section of the brain that told her to tense her muscle, but they forgot to turn it off. People struggling with this will become tense and cause themselves to walk lower to the ground, which in turn will force them to get a new center of gravity. So, when I was worried that my sister would fall over because of being off balance, I would force her to stand straight up. But that was the very thing that was causing her to be off balance. I had to learn to accept being bent over was a healthy and normal feature of the disease. You have to work with your loved one to help them get use to the new way of walking and getting around.

One thing I did learn is that when I could get her to be in a relaxed state, it was easier for her muscle to calm down and lighten up. One quick way to help her with this process was to reduce high-end stimuli, such as loud music and coffee. What I would use were soft lighting and soft music. The music seemed to penetrate any tension that was on her mind. You will find that calming music will be one of your biggest ally.

Visual – Auditory – Touch – Smell – Taste

Imagine, if you will, someone sneaking into your house in the middle of the night and while you are asleep, they re-wire your brain. Everything you used to do, you now have a different way of doing it. This idea is similar to what happens in the mind of someone with dementia because all of their senses are disrupted.

Sight becomes an issue because somewhere between stages two and three they will start to lose their depth perception. They will develop what is called binocular vision. The center of the brain that controls vision is affected by dementia, and many will lose their peripheral vision as it begins to narrow down to the point where they can only see what is directly in front of them. It will seem at times as if they are staring at you, but they are simply trying to make out what is in front of them. Over time, this will shift from binocular vision to monocular vision where they will see as a person who has a telescope up to their eye, but it is out of focus, and they cannot remove it. This will strongly impact their judgment of what they see in front of them. This is where you will have a lot of loved ones falling over because they cannot judge where they are walking or if they are going up or down a flight of stairs. I had a few occasions where my sister fell and badly bruised her face because she could not navigate a flight of stairs.

Over time, speech and hearing also became issues. Dementia generates what you may call white noise or sound distortions. With this going inside the heads of your loved one, it is as if you are speaking to them while in the middle of a windstorm. Your voice has to fight to be heard amongst the other words and sounds they hear from within their head. This will impact not only their hearing, but also what they are saying. It is kind of on the same level of a person giving a speech and in the middle of their presentation a marching band bursts in and plays music that is loud and strong and throws the speech presenter off while in the middle of their presentation.

Because my sister's for vision was becoming more and more distorted, she had to learn to compensate how her brain took in the information. Touch became a major key player. She would pick up and touch objects and examine the feel and texture of everything. Her brain was constantly telling her that she was cold, so she always wanted a coat or sweater on. It did not matter if the temperature was 95 degrees out and sweat was pouring off her, she, for comfort sake, had to have a sweater or coat on, or she would make everyone else's lives miserable. One of the other disadvantages of her skin's sensitivity was that when sores developed— unless it were infected and extremely painful—it would sometimes go unnoticed. Also, when it came to the loss of bodily function, my sister lost the means to sense when she was urinating or how uncomfortable it made her body feel to have urine against her skin.

As the disease progressed, my sister's sense of smell began to diminish. She could not distinguish if a smell were pleasant or repulsive. She could not tell if she was dirty and had an odor coming off of her. To talk to her about taking a shower was a difficult process at times. She hated taking showers and grew quite a resistance to the process because it was too confusing, and she hated getting help because she felt embarrassed that she needed that level of help to get things done.

Finally, I also began to notice that my sister's taste complex changed. My sister, before this disease, was overweight for much of her life. But there was a period where she because a health nut. She would eat extremely healthy, well-balanced diets. No sweets, and no red meats. Well, after dementia kicked in, it was as if much of the conscious thinking around healthy eating drifted away. She developed a taste for red meat and especially sweet foods. It got to a point that if she did not get anything sweet on her plate, she would refuse to eat.

Medication adjustment

When I got involved with taking care of my sister, I knew she was having some blood pressure issues, and she was taking medication to help address that. When we started managing her care, we started her on two of the leading brands of medication that most doctors know to prescribe. *Aricept* (donepezil) and *Namenda* (memantine) are the leading drugs on the market. They each came with their side effects. The combination brought on nausea, headaches and confusion. With these side effects, we had to add two other medications to control mood swings and sleep disorders. With the combination she was taking, she began to have muscle aches and seizure-like symptoms. This then caused us to add on two other types of medication. She then developed muscle stiffness, which led to a muscle relaxer.

Overall, the point I am trying to make here is that sometimes medication is not always the best way, and you have to weigh the cause and effects before you begin any medication. For dementia, the medication does not fix it only adjusts the behavior that the caregiver is having trouble managing. By taking this approach, versus equipping yourself to respond better, you now have created a situation where the medication can do more harm than good for your loved one.

Over time there is more dementia and less them

Let me start by stating the obvious: doctors are working with full intensity to find a cure and daily treatments for dementia. However, what has been developed so far is limited in how it can help. We as caregivers/partners are faced with how we are going to choose to address this disease. Time will become both our friend and our enemy. Depending on the stage you discover your loved one has this disease, and how you work with them to adjust their lifestyle, will determine the time and quality of life you will have. This disease forces you to cherish time and to consider mortality. This disease slowly strips away memory, personality, kindness, and makes you and you loved one vulnerable.

As the disease grows, it will consume and take time, energy, money, love, peace, comfort and convenience. Each day, you will have to say goodbye to your loved one in areas of their life. You must come to place where you understand that they will never get back. And yet, you will still have to function and be a rock for them to lean on and look to daily. You have to come to terms that each day there will be more dementia and less them.

What you are experiencing will cause you to adjust how you love and will be able to show your expression. It is emotionally painful to know that your loved one no longer recognizes you. You then have to re-introduce yourself to them. After a while, you simply become that nice person that comes to see them every day. As you go through this, you will find it is very easy to get bitter over the hand that life has dealt you. I felt that as well, and the bitterer I got, the more I began to write. I was not going to let this disease steal from me and get to have the final victory. I wanted to help my sister's life mean something. That is why I write. I wanted people to get to know her. I wanted to give people hope to find a way to be at peace with what they are experiencing and to find a means to move forward with a healthy level of confidence.

Mouth sensory

This was not an issue my sister had, but after talking to other families with loved ones with this issue, I have heard stories of how they would take foreign items and place them in their mouths. As a warning, you almost have to childproof their living environment and be mindful of items they could place in their mouth. As they progress through the disease, their mouth becomes an alternate sensory processing area. They place things in their mouth to establish a sense of security and fulfill the minds natural curiosity. So do not be surprised if you see this occur, just take precautions.

Fighting for freedom

There were a couple of situations where my sister became combative. This is very common with people with an advanced stage of dementia. It was shocking to see much of it play out. My sister, for the most part, was a very deliberate type of person. She knew what she wanted and worked hard to get things done. She hated being told what to do. For her to be placed in a position where she had to be under authority was a hard thing for her to face. So, when she was having trouble with processing instructions, and the people providing the instructions were being direct and /or pushy, it would trigger a harsh reaction from my sister and then the person giving the instruction would insist even more. All of this caused my sister to escalate into violence as a means to defend herself from people trying to force her to do what they wanted to do.

I have to note, I personally never had that issue with my sister, except when I had to intervene with her and another caregiver who was trying to give her bad directions. Primarily, I had to learn how to read my sister's body language, and I learned how to adjust her frame or reference to make it easier for her to cooperate with what I was assisting her to do. The key word here is "assist." What I was doing was creating a mental partnership where she could feel like she was in charge, but I would plant mental seeds in her head that were directing her with what I needed her to do. It required patience and a lot of creativity, but it worked very effectively.

Keep memories positive

This will become one of your most powerful allies and bring so much peace to your family environment. One of the things that my sister would do, when her vision was still good, was walk around the house and look for photos and take them back to her room and hide them in her bed. What she was doing was trying to fight to hang on to memories. The photos functioned as a memory anchor.

What works very effectively is to collect photos, family videos, and audio that are meaningful to them. The larger the photo, the better, especially as their vision fades, because it will make it easier for them to see. The photos will allow them to drift back to a place of peace. If you can, encourage family members and friends to record things in video or audio form, and compile it in a way where you can play it back for them on a regular basis. It will create a powerful environment for comfort. You will find that you can manage their care with a lot less medication if you can control their stress. The memory enhancement helps in a huge way.

Live in the general, not in the specifics

In our positive and progressive world, we are conditioned to get on some agenda and to meet some goal. We are told to fight hard and press ahead, to build, and to grow and develop. We like to work things down to minor detail. However, the perspective of a person with dementia goes through some changes that at times is frightening to them and confusing to caregivers. Things that were important to them become not so important anymore. They lose their concern for fitting into society. Their passions become very simplified. Some simple things become the staple of their day. What helps, in the dynamics of a healthy relationship, is as a caregiver, to seriously and with full intent, back off of pushing to get it right and stick to high-end agendas. If you want to care for someone with dementia, you have to be willing to let go of agendas and learn how to read the signs and just go with the flow of life.

Be a detective, not a judge

You are going to discover some things about your loved one. You will be placed in a position where you will have to dig through the details of their life. You will find out things that you did not want to know. I am not going to get into the deep detail of my sister's life, but what I am going to say, is when you find out things about people, it is a natural temptation to pass judgment over how they chose to live their life in the past and how they are living today. To a degree, certain things need to be discovered, but the major temptation will be to fight the strong urge to pass judgment. Most people do this so often when it comes to practically everyone, that we do it without thinking. However, passing judgment will create barriers, and it increases stress between you and the one you are going to care for. You have to be willing to find personal liberty in choosing to not hold things against them or to use whatever you find out as some evidence to condemn them to a position of guilt and shame. The results will more than likely lead to them fighting back in a non-rational way.

Hygiene

This next section is an important one because it deals with dignity and sensitivity for your loved one, as well as for yourself. I want you to take a few minutes and think slowly and methodically. You are lying in your bed and are alone and asleep. The next thing you know, someone comes into your room and tells you to get up because they are going to have you take a shower. First of all, you are taken by surprise. Who is this and how dare they come into your room and disrupt your peaceful sleep? They come in and start giving you orders. Then they have the gall to walk over to you and place their hands on your body and to even go as far as starting to undress you.

For a person with dementia, this is where it gets real touchy. When it comes to people undressing them, it either means one of two things to them: either they feel attacked or that someone intends to have sex with them. Some with dementia interpret that as a good thing or bad, based on what thoughts may have been flowing through their mind at the time. So, my first recommendation is to slow down and watch the approach.

Bathing

If you are going to bathe them, the first thing you will need to do is gain their permission and use persuasion to get them to feel as if it was their idea that they are taking a bath. Be gentle and clear with them in your approach. Always establish eye contact whenever possible. Speak softly to them, and remember to smile as you talk. This will bring down their guard. Always make the first touch to them be a handshake. At that point, gently hold on to their hand and caress it. You should get them to start talking about their day, and speak regarding some special event coming up and how great it would be if they got cleaned up for it. This would require you to really get to know their likes and dislikes. You may want to plan bathing time before a special event. My sister loved to go to church. So it was easy to get her to take a shower before church. It would make her feel extra special to get up and prepped for this event. In my case, I had to utilize the help of my wife to help her bathe. I wanted to make sure I did not create any embarrassing situations for her. I wanted her to feel that her dignity was being protected all the time. I wanted her to feel that I valued her time and opinion. I would ask her opinion, and I would give her choices and preferences.

One other thing to note, because a person with dementia is not conscious of how much they drink and the hygiene is lacking, their skin can become very dry and sensitive. Make sure to use mild soaps and warm water. Also, assist them with the lotion process. This will prevent dry and cracking skin from developing.

Bed wetting

This was a tough area for me to deal with. My sister was very particular about her bed and bedding. She insisted on staying in her queen-sized bed, with her large comforters, and tons of pillows. However, over time, the work to maintain her bedding became too mentally complicated for her. What I mean by that is, that her pillows and blankets had detailed patterns on them. This visual effect caused my sister to get confused to the point as to how to get out of bed. She would get wrapped in her blankets and then before she knew it; she would wet her bed.

That was a learning experience. It taught me that even if you are dealing with a strong willed person, you have to take a leadership role and make some executive decision on how you will arrange things to provide good and reasonable care. First of all, it will become critical that you simplify and de-clutter their lifestyle. They may resist at times, but you have to find a way to do this sooner rather than later. When it comes to the size of bed they are in, you may want to go down to a twin sized bed. It will be easier for them to manage and navigate. Based on their condition and mobility, you may want to check with your resources and acquire a hospital grade bed.

Well before the incontinence starts, you will want to use bed padding and a leak proof covering over your mattress. Believe me, once urine is inside a mattress, it does not come out. So, to protect your mattress, and other furniture, as well as your loved one's skin, get the covering.

Next, you will want to consider utilizing adult diapers. They have some cool brands out now that do not even look like diapers. Some look like fancy underwear, especially the brand that they make for ladies. You will want to ask your loved ones to try out the new underwear so that they can see how comfortable they feel. If you can get them sold on the comfort and style, they will feel more apt to cooperate. If you push, they will resist. Above all, you do not want this to turn into an embarrassing situation for them. Fight to preserve their dignity and ask their preference and seek their cooperation and offer them suggestions and alternatives that work best for both of you. There will be a lot of trial and error, but if you keep at it, you can develop and a win-win situation for both of you.

Understanding the stages of grief

In 1969, Elizabeth Kubler-Ross published a book that many in the psychology world use to help those that are dealing with loss and grief. That book is called "On Death and Dying." This is a very well written and informative book. It gives an insight of what all humans and even other animal types deal with emotionally when facing some loss. There are five major stages, and there is no specific sequence nor is there a particle amount of time a person may spend in each. Also, a person transitions from one to the other so fast it may seem like they have not gone through a particle stage. The stages are, and in no particular order, denial, anger, bargaining, depression and acceptance.

Denial and isolation

To hear that you are suspected to have dementia, especially with all the media and information out there about it, you could easily feel like someone has kicked the legs right out from under you. You do not want to hear it from your doctor, family or friends. You try to resume your life as if nothing is wrong. You isolate yourself from people and things that could remind you that this disease could ever exist within you. Just like the person with dementia, you as the caregiver can face this as well. You do not want to hear that your mom, dad, sister, brother or even child has such a serious disease. This may have been a person you have come to rely on, but now the roles have to switch. That can be emotionally devastating. You are forced to ask the question, "How could this be?" The search could leave you feeling broken and helpless because there is no reasonable answer for how and why.

Anger

After you come to grips that you have dementia, or you are in a position where you have to care for someone with dementia, here is where things could get rough. You might start to ask yourself "why me?" "What did I do to deserve this disease?" A person can become so enraged that they could do harm to themselves, or others. They may also do something with their financial and legal status. I have heard of cases, where some, as a way of dealing with the pain, go on a spending spree as if this was it for them; so they wanted to live it up before their memory was gone. Others have gotten into fights or committed violent acts or engaged in an activity where they knew harm would come to them. These are signs to be aware of so if you know your loved one has been given the news of the diagnosis, it will help you with protecting their well-being. Family counseling for you and your loved one will aid you in the grieving process if you feel it is getting out of control. Another good idea after the initial shock has set in, is to have the loved one sit with the doctor. Along with a caregiver or another family member, have the doctor explain what they suspect about what they found and to lay out what to expect the patient to experience over the course of the disease. Also, you will ask the doctor to lay out a treatment plan and alternatives, as well as proposed expectation for each type of treatment.

Bargaining

The natural inclination is to question why and ask a lot of "What if ...?" type questions: "What did I do to cause this? What could I have done differently? What could I do to reverse the damages? I am young and have so much life ahead of me. There has to be another way?" Some will openly, or in secret, make deals with God with hope for a reversal or for this disease to pass, versus accepting and treating it in a healthy manner.

Depression

Depression can be expressed in a few different ways. Some will express their depression in a loud and vocal manner, and you can hear it and see it on their face and expression. Others are quiet and reserved. The first thing we have to back away from is labeling it as being wrong to be depressed. The effective tactful thing to do, if you are the caregiver, is to be there and present. Questions will arise. It is all right if you do not have all the answers, but you can partner with your loved one to seek good answers and to ask a series of better questions. It is important to help your loved one ask descriptive questions. These might include: "What do I need to expect will happen to me over the next few months?"; "How will this affect my ability to do my job?"; "What holistic measures can I take that will support my memory?"" "Since some of my memory cells have died, is there a way I can build new memory cells that can keep me going and functioning that will enable me to learn?" That last question may not have a good answer, but every doctor has to be on the lookout on how to give an answer to such a question.

Acceptance

For some, acceptance comes long and far off. A person dealing with dementia may not even experience this until it is too late to establish a quality life base. It will take a patient, loving and persistent caregiver to help their loved one navigate this path of life. You may have entered this stage of care in the 5th stage of dementia, at which point you are limited in how you can relate. However, you can at least work at aiding them at preserving their remaining dignity. Based on your loved one's personality, they may still need and crave social interaction, and others would prefer to be left alone to just a few loved ones. It is important to establish an atmosphere of peace for them, as well as yourself. There is a huge difference between what is perceived to be right and what is right based on whole health. A person could receive the best and a ton of medical attention, but that may erode them mentally. It is important to examine where your loved one is at and where you are at as a caregiver and work at establishing a happy medium.

Get a good assessment of the type of dementia

There is a very high risk of getting the wrong diagnosis. We all have to understand that our bodies are designed to last a long time and that they are pre-designed to function in a healthy way. If treated with care, we could get great usage from it. It is a balanced system. If we do anything in excess, we could inadvertently cause damage. With this in mind, we have to understand how the majority of doctors are trained. They are taught to understand our body makeup and functionality. You have to respect what it takes to become that knowledgeable. Some doctors push their training to a certain degree that simply by looking at you and asking a few good questions they can determine that a rash you have came from a new fabric softener you just started using. However, there are also doctors how have mastered medicines. Not to say that medicines are bad, but if a doctor does a quick examination of you and starts prescribing medication for you, as opposed to you changing your lifestyle, then you may want to speak up and ask for a time out, rewind the tape and ask deeper question as to why they are suggesting the route they chose and ask about alternatives.

It is extremely important that you get a clear diagnosis of what type of dementia your loved one may have. It is important you put together a strategy of how you plan on treating it at each stage. You need to talk to the doctor up front about how often they need to see your loved one and what type of things they will be assessing. You need to get a list of things you as a care provider need to stay aware of and what to chart and document. You will want to keep a good log of what you are experiencing. This will be a powerful tool to help your doctor do a better job of prescribing care and recommendation of better care for your loved one. You will want to get a medical referral to a neurological specialist as well as a psychologist that specializes in coping with individuals and families with dementia. Dementia attacks the mind, body, and spirit of the individual as well as it can erode the safety, security, and foundation of any strong family. To get a good idea of what you are dealing with will help you defend against the worst that could happen, and it will enable you to redefine what "worst" looks like.

Push for a PET scan and then pursue a gradual adjustment of the drugs

Positioning Emission Tomography (PET) is a scan that produces a 3D image of the area of the body that they are trying to diagnose. It uses radioactive tracer dyes that map out blood flow and muscle, tissue, and bone structure. It is especially good for detecting metabolism (how your body uses sugar), which is extremely important when it comes to determining which section of the brain is functional and which have died off.

Because it is nuclear medicine, there are risks involved. Any person who is pregnant or thinks they may be pregnant should not do this test. A person will be administered the dye a period before the test via intravenously or ingestion or by gas. After absorption, they will be taken to a testing area. During the process, they will lay in specialized bed. The bed is on a track that slides onto a dark cylinder. They will be instructed to remain still during this process. This test will prove to be valuable in determining the stage the dementia patient is in and what to expect over time. If the test is given more than once, it will help to gauge how fast the disease is progressing along. Based on that information, it will be a wonderful tool to help you adjust any medication your loved one may be on or which medications to wean them off of.

Aricept and Namenda have about a two-year span on what it does in the system

The two leading drugs to help with sustaining a quality of life for your loved are *Aricept* and *Namenda*. There are some important things you need to know concerning these and others that are on the market. You should also be aware of other studies that are taking place that may impact future medicines.

Aricept (generic: *Donepezil*) comes from the cholinesterase inhibitors family. Others that are in that same family are *Exelon* (generic: *Rivastigmine*) and *Razadyne* (generic: *Galantamine*). *Aricept* is the leading drug on the market and can be taken from early onset all the way to severe levels of dementia. *Exelon* and *Razadyne* should only be prescribed for mild to moderate levels of dementia. This medication helps addresses issues with memory loss, confusion, and problems with thinking and reasoning. The way it works is it prevents the breakdown of chemical messengers that transports memory information. That messenger is called, acetylcholine (a-SEA-til-KOH-lean). The effective range of these medicines will get you a delay in the decline of the memory of about six to twelve months. It is not designed to be taken as a long term solution. All of these medicines carry the same side effects, which are, nausea, vomiting, loss of appetite, and increased frequency of bowel movements.

As a patient moves into a moderate level, doctors have been known to get good results by combining *Aricept* along with *Namenda* (generic: *Memantine*).

This medication helps to improve memory, attention, reason, language, and the ability to perform simple tasks. It regulates the activity of glutamate, a different messenger chemical involved in learning and memory. When combined with a cholinesterase, it greatly sustains the performance of the cognitive skills. The side effects are a headache, constipation, confusion, and dizziness.

Vitamin E, also known as alpha-tocopherol, is an antioxidant. Antioxidants may protect brain cells and other body tissues from certain kinds of chemical wear and tear. However, there is limited research information on how well this performs, and if you are going to use this as your treatment, you need to make sure it is closely monitored by your doctor.

No matter what medication or natural remedy you choose for your loved one to take, please keep a log of what is used and how often it is issued. Monitor what side effects they are getting and make sure you provide that detail to the doctor at the regular checkup. At that point, if you need to change anything, you can have accurate information as to what will be changed, but always, ask why they change and what medication they would alternatively recommend. You want to get into questions related to the combination of the medication and what the mixture will produce by way of side effects. That way you will know if it is worth it to make the medication change.

Also, I am going to recommend that if you have a loved one that is at an early stage in the disease, please contact the Alzheimer's Association and try to get placed on a case study. The information they can gain from your record keeping and what treatment your loved one is getting could lead to a better treatment plan for them as well as improve their quality of life. Above all, by doing this, you are pushing doctors to find a cure faster. So make the call today.

Diet and exercise

No matter what is going wrong with you, no matter what you are going to see the doctor for, they will always tell you that you need to eat a better diet and to exercise. If you are overweight, diet and exercise. If you have diabetes, diet and exercise. If you break your leg, diet and exercise.

When it comes to dementia, you want to put emphasis on this. My suggestion for this would be to get your loved one on a diet that is high in fiber and low in fat. I recommend, and so do many doctors, to make sure to get six to eight servings of fruit or vegetables daily. Consider reducing the amount of protein you are getting from red meats. Get your starches from whole grain, and drink plenty of water. By doing this, you can better regulate the types of protein you are getting into your body, and you will help your body metabolize sugar in a more refined manner and help better fuel your brain. Also, you may want to consider taking Omega-3 in the form of fish oil pills. This works great with helping to manage the cholesterol.

When it comes to exercise, if you are dealing with a person who has never exercised or is physically incapable of exercise, this can be a little more challenging to accomplish. You should find something they can manage and would love to do. If you could do it with them, it would be an opportunity for bonding and health for both of you. For a person dealing with dementia, it is extremely important you get them to engage in something cardiovascular based; walking, riding, running or anything along those lines.

This will increase the flow of oxygenated blood to the brain. This will help with metabolizing sugars that are within the blood stream, which is the food that your brain needs to process at its best.

Coconut Oil

According to the researchers at greenmedinfo.com, "The rationale for using coconut oil as a potential AD [Alzheimer's Disease] therapy is related to the possibility that it could be metabolized to ketone bodies that would provide an alternative energy source for neurons, and thus compensate for mitochondrial dysfunction." The researchers proposed that ketone bodies formed as a byproduct of coconut oil metabolism might offset Aβ-induced impairment of mitochondrial function and thus energy metabolism.

I know that this is a lot of technical jargon, and by no means am I claiming to be smarter than those in the medical field researching all these cures. What I am stating is that when you are caring for your loved one and see them slowly slip away, it hurts deeply. You become desperate and will try practically anything and everything to try to get them back to a healthy state. Beside coconut oil, there are other alternative treatments, but no matter what route you choose, try to weight the pros and cons of every treatment against the quality of life you are trying to achieve with your loved one, along with the quality life you need to have balanced for yourself.

Chapter 7 - Early Responses and Lifestyle Adjustment

"Life is change. Growth is optional. Choose wisely."
– Unknown

There is an old saying that goes: "It's not what happens to you as much as it is how you respond to what happens to you that determines how thing will turn out." The reason you picked up this book is because you needed help and answers. You gravitated to this book, in particular, because you connected with someone who has lived through this disease. You keep reading because you believe there are some great tools in this book that will enable you to give greater care along with placing an emphasis on caring for yourself. Well, I am not going to disappoint you. What I found is that when I started this process, I did not do enough research, and I did not seek out enough help. If I had done that right out of the gate, I could have made a better life condition for my total family make up, so that I could care for my sister and not destroy the stability of my family dynamics.

Changing the lifestyle plan

Many people have not considered this, but we all have a lifestyle plan. Some have gone as far as to write it down and share it with family members to have means to communicate what is valuable to them. But like any plan, it may have to change. When it comes to caring for someone with Alzheimer's or dementia you have to come to terms that his or her lifestyle plan will change as well as yours. The sooner you find the disease along with the current health status determines the rate of change. You have to take into account what kind of life they used to have and then help them restructure a new plan that is more comfortable and fitting for where they are today. Moreover, you will have to adjust that plan over time.

You also have to look at your current status as a caregiver. Are you working or are you unemployed? Do you have a lot of free time or will you need help to come in and work with you? Are you caring for small children while caring for your loved one with the disease? Are you married to your loved one? Was your loved one the primary bread winner? How busy of a lifestyle did you have, and are you ready to slow things down? Overall, you have to look at your lifestyle and map out what you may expect. This will help you make a determination of what you will hang onto and what you will have to let go. But, either way, you have to come to terms with the fact that change will come in some way. You have to decide how you will master the change.

Building a strong support team

You are going to find that if you can build a strong support tem, you will make a huge improvement in the quality of care provided for your loved one and help to preserve your peace of mind. There are a lot of people that you can incorporate into your team. It will require some planning and tact on your part to build the best team.

One of the first people to start with is your loved one's doctor. This is the person you want to work with to develop your medical blueprint on how to holistically treat the impact of the disease. Your doctor can help answer a lot of questions as well as give you a medical referral to a specialist; your doctor's input will help the other doctors make a better decision.

Next, you will want to talk to all your close family and friends. That could be the sibling, parents, and children of your loved one. It is vital for you not to keep this to yourself. There are dangers involved. One of the families that I did research included a married woman acquired dementia and her husband who was her caregiver. They both lead a simple and quiet life. The husband worked very hard not to embarrass his wife, and so he kept it secret to all of their family and friends that she was ill. After about three years of care, the husband died of a heart attack. The couple had children who were all in different states. When they came back home for the funeral, was when they discovered that something was not right with their mom. The family was already in a tailspin from losing their husband and father, but they were also thrust into a care plan for their mom that none of them was prepared to address. This is why it is very important that a caregiver develops a plan that deliberately includes the help of others and to plan ahead, so that if something were to happen to the primary caregiver, to the point that they could not fulfill their duties, they would have someone who could step in and help out.

Do not be afraid to include the help of friends, especially those with religious affiliations to organizations or clubs. I would recommend that if they are affiliated with some kind of church, you try to take some time and meet with the leadership of that organization and let them know how they can help. Help could come in the form of making them a meal, or simply sitting with them and talking about the good old days. Please bear in mind that what you ask for in the way of help today may change in roles over time. I know that while I was growing up, the church I attended had a group of people who dedicated time and resources to outreach and shut-in visitation. They would regularly go and visit the seniors and disabled that were members of our church. I highly recommend that you tap into this resources and bring them into your support team.

If you live on a street with and are connected with your neighbors, it would be a great idea to inform your neighbors of your loved one's condition and give them your number. You should at least ask them to be a second pair of eyes for you, and if they see your loved one walk off from the neighborhood or attempt to take off in the family car, they could alert you so you can take appropriate action. They could also act as an emergency backup in the event you need some quick help for having someone temporary look after your loved one.

You will also want to talk to your local police and fire department and alert them to the fact that your loved one has dementia. Find out if they have some sort of Silver Alert program put in place just in case your loved one goes missing. You will want them to have a recent picture of your loved one in the event that they will need to do a quick neighborhood search or all-points bulletin.

Once you get your boots on the ground, you will want to expand your net. What I mean by that is taking advantage of the net. If you live in a community where you have connections with people in your neighborhood, and especially if you have a Facebook group, by all means tap in and use it. You will want to make sure to use this to keep up to date with community events, but you can also use this as a low-level alert system, in the event your loved one goes missing. You could easily post a picture of your loved one with a quick notation about who they are and explain that they are under your care and are battling with dementia. You would be surprised how fast and effective this works, and how it will help you reconnect with your wondering loved one.

While you are online, I highly recommend that you visit the Alzheimer's Association website. You will find a wealth of resources there. This is an organization that has a national reach on everything related to finding a cure for Alzheimer's as well as helping people understand the impact this disease has taken on our society. They have developed a great network that is plugged into practically every community and that has helped with locating doctors and specialist. They aid the caregiver by getting them connected with support groups and educational resources. They also run a wide variety of case studies that help find better treatments and, Lord willing, a cure for the disease. They can prove to be one of your greatest allies.

Beyond the help of your family doctor, you will need to get your loved one connected with a great neurologist. This is a person that you as a caregiver will also want to get to know. You will want to know their background with treating patients with dementia. What I mean by that is, you need to ask them how many patients have they treated within the past ten years, and what kind of variations of this disease they have treated. You want to know if they offer, along with medication, any form of therapeutic holistic treatment for the patient. Some doctors have a pattern of medication that they offer for the standard symptoms they see, and sit back and hope for the best, but that does not promote any balanced care for the patient or for you as a caregiver. Just like you are partnering in care for your loved one, you will need a neurologist that is patient about partnering with you to provide best care and information.

One thing that I have come to understand about neurologists is that because of a wide variety of issues that have impacted the brain and with all the studies taking place, they are extremely busy and hard to schedule their appointments.   If you live in a metropolitan area, odds are the doctor you get will be extremely busy and hard to see. So you will have to work diligently with your insurance company and, I would also recommend, try to get an alternative recommendation if you have a neurologist that has too high of a case load. Also, you want one that will sit down and talk with you and answer all of your questions. Be aware of doctors that do a quick work and basic cognitive testing and issue a script and sends you on your way. You need a doctor who is patient and passionate about the wellbeing of your loved one. If not, the impact of each progressive stage with be harder on your loved one. Stay observant and ask lots of questions to get the best out of the relationship you have with the neurologist.

Another team member to consider, especially if you are still working a job, is to incorporate the help of adult day care. I have to say, this proved one of the best experience I have ever had. The care place I found was phenomenal. The care leader of this facility was a registered nurse, and she hired the most loving and qualified staff. They were patient and caring and provided my sister the love and compassion she needed. They worked hard to protect my sister's dignity while giving direction and care. They set up family counseling that helped reinforce the strength and stability of the family unit. They enabled me to have a high level of trust that my sister was safe, cared for, and loved on. It enabled me to go to work in peace and put balance into my life. The director invested herself into the life of all the people that were under her care. Even when my sister had to go into a nursing home, she would come up and visit and give love encouragement. It brought joy to my heart, and I will forever appreciate the love and bonds created at the Auburn Hills Quality of Life Center, and my praise goes out to Jackie Smiertka.

The next member of your team to include will be a quality nursing home. This is a hard page to turn. A person has to have a balanced heart to face this level of reality. For some, this is coming to terms that things are beyond the level of help you are equipped to provide. What I can say is, when I got to this point, I was at my end and out of my depth. I did not know how to care for my sister anymore. I knew I had to get her in a nursing home, but I had no clue of the different types that are out there. There are some awesome places out there that I ran into that made me want to move in myself. I also visited some that I felt scared to walk even in the door. What I would recommend is that before you get to this stage, you should take some time and visit various homes that are in your area. You will want to look at the quality of care, as well as cost. You will want to compare value versus expense. As you walk the halls of the nursing home, pay attention to the smells and take a good look at the faces of the patients. This is something that is near and dear to me, and it is my aim that your loved one get the best in care and can live the highest quality of life. So, I am pleading with you to find a place that expresses *home*. There are nursing homes where the management and workers are there simply to get a paycheck. There is nothing wrong with a paycheck; there *is*, however, something wrong with being granted the responsibility to care for another human being and then to fail and neglect or give less than your best in care. Do your due diligence and look, ask questions, and pick a place that will protect, care, and provide not just a place to live but a place where they will receive love.

Another member to bring is your team is a family support group. I would start with any religious or social affiliate to see if there are any support groups available. Beyond that, ask your doctor or even the Alzheimer's Association to see if they know of any support groups in your area. The value of connecting with a group is it will give you another line of defense. You will have a team of people who are in the same boat as you. Some may be walking through a more advanced stage and others will be just joining as well. You will discover that you are not alone and that there is strength in numbers. You will encounter people who understand your situation. You will be given advice from those who have walked through and developed a wealth of hindsight that will become invaluable in the care you will provide. You will have a shoulder to cry on, and you will find that there are people you will encounter that can validate your feelings as well as sure up your heart as you face the trials ahead. Their insight will help you navigate the system, the red tape, and the snares that may lay ahead of you. It will be most effective if you can find the time to meet face-to-face with a group, but if you cannot, you could look for on-line groups. But it would be beneficial that you connect and never try to go it alone.

Another option is to include a wellness coach in your circle of support. This can be scary and challenging for some. It is not an easy to talk about your feelings or to have someone give you ideas and suggestions on how to live your life. A wellness coach is someone experienced with working with caregivers. You need someone who can be honest and forthright, and who can have good insight into family dynamics. You need someone who can be real and honest and let you know when you are giving the care in an unhealthy manner. That second pair of eyes could mean the difference between a broken life or one filled with dignity and hope.

Home healthcare supplies

If you live near any major metropolitan area, you should be able to find a local supplier of adult healthcare resources with minimal effort. There are some items you may need that may be of value to you, based on the condition of your loved one. You will find, if you are ordering consumables goods, sites that offer a discount to order in bulk, such as bedding pads and adult diapers.

I want you to think in terms as if you were an expecting parent of a newborn. Think regarding bedding, clothing, transportation safety, and feeding. If you had a newborn, you would first think of where you would place them. Will your loved one be able to sleep in a standard bed or will you need to consider an adjustable hospital bed? Bear in mind that over time, your loved will become incontinent. So, the mattress type matters greatly. You want to have one that is water resistant. If your loved one is in a king sized bed, starting out, your will want to consider transitioning down to a medical twin sized bed. The bigger bed leads to confusion for the loved one as time progresses. If your loved one is prone to falling out of bed, there are railing systems you can add to a standard bed, or you can get a hospital bed with rails. Also, if they are prone to falling, you can get an audible fall alert for the bed and any chairs or wheelchairs.

As far as transportation, if your loved one can walk, I would recommend a cane, but not a walker. If it is mechanical, over time, they will lose their ability to remember how to operate it, or ever forget it when going out. What I recommend is to adjust the furniture in the home so that everything is within a few feet of each other. That way they will have something to hang onto when working. This reduces the risk of confusion and falling more than a walker would. If they are having a particularly hard time walking, and you have to go out a lot, you should consider getting a lightweight, portable wheelchair.

In the bathroom, you will want to get a shower chair, and on the toilet, you will need to install falling rails if your loved one has that problem. You will also want to invest in a senior monitor that receives audio and video so you can monitor when they are in their room. Another item to consider is a Wi-Fi camera for common areas in and outside of your home. That way, you can monitor when you have to leave your loved one for any period. One other source is to consider is craigslist. There are a ton of resources out there that you will find some people practically giving away. Do not be afraid to investigate this resource. This is a short list of items, and I will cover more items later in this book, as well on my blog site. If you have questions about anything listed, please feel free to check out the site *CourageousCaregiver.org* and I will be happy to address any of your concerns.

Managing outside help and loved ones
When it comes to this topic, you have to be willing to take on the role of project manager. Just like in any company or organization, if there is ever a major project taking place, it is usually headed up by a project manager. They manage resources in the way of people, time, and expenses. As a project manager, you have to keep your finger on the pulse of everything that is taking place with your loved one and not only manage schedules and their health, but you also have to stay tuned to your available resources and through quality communication, direct them to how to best help you. Please bear in mind that, over time, you will lose resources, and it is of no fault of their own. It is just the nature of people's passion for doing long-term care. You must be creative and deliberate in continuously seeking out new resources to add to your team and split the load. You will have to get creative with how you incorporate your resources so as to not to burn them out too quickly. Also, learn and master the power of gratitude. People love to hear 'Thank You," and "I appreciate all the ways that you help." It goes a long

way and helps brighten someone else's day. You will find that the better you are at recruiting help, the easier it becomes to make your dollars stretch with what you will need to support your loved one.

They need assurance that they are not going crazy

As a person progresses through dementia, they naturally feel scared or as if they are losing their mind. In a way, they are, but in the bigger scheme of things, they, like anyone else, are fighting and coming to terms with the fact they are no longer in control of their life. They do not know who to trust and, at times, they cannot even trust themselves. Their stress level will run high. You have to stay aware that all of this is taking place and actively engage them in an atmosphere of peace and assurance that they will be safe, loved, and under great care. Practice smiling. What you project will reflect. If you are at peace, you have a greater means of influencing peace within your loved one. If you are sure and confident, then they will respect that and be more willing to place their trust in your hands. Be deliberate about getting you and all of your support team on the same page. As the disease progresses, the page of life will turn, but by using this guide, you can manage your stress because you know what is on the next page. Knowing what to expect makes the transition that much easier.

Chapter 8 - Support Resources

"Don't look down on anyone unless you're helping them up." – Lyndon B. Johnson

Applying for aid and financial support

Some people, a rare few, have done an awesome job with planning ahead for their future and care while their prognosis is still in the early stages, and had an idea of how they wanted care provided and by whom. There are those that made wise investments where money is a non-issue. They have set-up medical insurance and have a great family doctor that they have seen for years. Some have even gone so far as to having a sit-down talk with who would be giving care and spelling out what it would look like up until they take their last breath on this side of life. It is my prayer that you have ended up with that person, and if that is the case, you can toss this book in the trash or pass it on to someone else who may need it. But my bet is, you are reading this book because that is not the case. You are over your head and out of your depth with what you are facing, and you need help and need it now. My heartfelt prays are with you, and I promise to pour out my best advice and research to help you get all the tools you need to be successful.

If placed in a position where you have to scramble and tap into resources, then one of your main resources will be financial support. I want you to put on your accountant hat at this time. You will have to create a means of checks and balance and high accountability for managing finances. To some, it may seem valiant to take it on the chin and dig deep into your own personal pockets and come up with resources to help take care of your loved one. However, as selfish as it seems, you will want to use your personal finances as the last resort. You will need to track everything that happens to your loved one's assets and keep those assets separate from your own. You will also want to get a good snapshot of the status of their assets. You need to inventory all their possessions and try to come up with an assessed value for everything they own. You will want to distinguish between liquid and other. Based on what assets they have to manage, you then will need to consider how you are going to tactfully use their assets to cover the expenses of their needs. It will be difficult, but you will need to liquidate assets to get them in a usable form to take care of their medical and personal needs. As you are for them, you will need to track your expenses for what is required to take care of them. Track every cent. The reason I say this is because if you have to apply for conservatorship, your probate court will require a full account and an annual review of their status. Either way, you will need to get a good picture of what you are dealing with financially. Get it all on paper. If you can do this, it will prove to be valuable when dealing with any federal, state, or county agencies for coordinated care.

SSI - Disability

When your loved starts to show signs of dementia, especially if they are pre-retirement age, you will want to consider strongly applying for Social Security Income in the form of Disability. You can start the process by going to *http://www.ssa.gov/disabilityssi/apply.html*. Here you can find out the rules and requirement of who can apply. They are going to need a lot of detailed information on your loved one. I recommend that you apply on your loved one's behalf. They are going to ask a lot of detailed information about medical issues and treatment, as well as a lot of detail about their assets and their usage. This income is based on what assets the person may have as well as their condition and age. Now, sad to say, but I have seen a lot of cases where a person may apply and the claim is denied. Then usually within 60 days they are eligible to apply again. I have seen improved statics for getting helped and accepted is if a person uses an experienced SSI attorney. If you have a well-documented case and have done a good job of the accounting, ask around in your local support groups to see who has filed and has used a good attorney and see if you can retain their services. That way, you can get it pushed through on the first time out. It is not a lot of money, but if your loved one is entitled to it, then by all means, make sure they get it. Once again, the federal government wants you to do a good accounting of how that money is spent. You will want to set up a separate account in advance and, when applying for the funds, provide the routing number and account number so that the checks can be direct deposited. You will have to make an annual report of how the money is used, so take good notes.

Pension fund - early retirement

Pension? What is that? Well, believe it or not, some companies still have these. What has replaced these are 401K and IRA's. Either way, if your loved one has been documented as having dementia, and they are going through the disability process, many human resources departments have rules and provisions to set up an early issue of retirement funds as a means to subsidize someone with a terminal illness. Also, once you get a conservatorship, you can then talk to your loved one's financial institution about setting up payment of any IRA's. You can push to get all the money in one lump sum, or you can do an estimated dividend payment. I would take the monthly payout simply because if you have caught the disease early enough; you will need that continuous dispersant to last your loved one throughout the term of the disease. Once again, you will want to keep this money separated from your personal money, and you will want to give a full accounting of where every penny is spent.

Medicare

Medicare is supplemental medical insurance that you would normally get if you were of retirement age. You would get this issued from the former employer of your loved one. If they previously had a company issued insurance, being diagnosed with a medical disability would make them eligible for Medicare. You will need to work with their former human resources department. That is the procedure you need to follow if they are below retirement age. If they are above retirement age, then you can apply via *http://www.ssa.gov/medicare/apply.html*. If you have private insurance, then Medicare Part A and Part B can work alongside your plan. It would be a great idea to apply for this along with your disability and with luck, you will get the same caseworker for each and this will give you a central focal point for a person to work with.

Medicaid

If you are getting close to what they call a "spend down" in finical assets of your loved one, where you have their monthly balance less than approximately $2,000, then your loved one qualifies for Medicaid. Usually, that is the only stipulation that is given to delay getting Medicaid. In my sister's case, when she got to the end stage in her dementia, we had to submit a case quickly after we had admitted her to the hospital. Based on her income, she was above the speed down amount, so what was worked out was out of any monthly bill submitted by the hospital or by the nursing home, we had to spend out of her disability and retirement fund first, and if there was anything remaining on the bill, then Medicaid would cover the rest. This is why it is really important to pay close attention to any assets and develop a plan on how you liquidate any of those resources and use those fund to cover medical care. Please bear in mind that Medicaid and Medicare only cover related medical expenses, and when the federal government does a review of any assets your loved one has, they will be asking how assets are being spent for medical care. So, if any of the assets is being used to pay for anything else, that total sum will not be calculated in the spend down. In my sister's case, a portion of her disability was going toward paying for outstanding bills she had. Once she became eligible for Medicaid, I was no longer allowed to use her assets to cover her non-medical bills. All assets then become focused purely on medical care at that point.

Disability insurance

There is life, health, auto, and home insurance, however, a lot of people have not considered investing in disability insurance. It costs very little but has a high return. This is something you as a caregiver should consider getting for yourself. It could mean the difference between survivability and bankruptcy. If you are the major breadwinner for your family, please consider getting this so you can bring peace of mind to your spouse and family. It is an insurance plan that will pay out on a regular basis and sustain you and your family when you cannot work. What does this mean for your loved one who has the disease? When reviewing their assets, you will want to connect with their former HR department to see if they activated and applied for this insurance and find out who manages the disbursement. Find out what needs to be done to activate this.

Community awareness

Do you know your community and community leaders? Have you touched based with your local community center to see if they have a division that supports senior needs? Who can you talk to about senior care support groups? Have you checked the phone book or the internet to see if there are any adult senior care facilities around? If so, can you make contact with them to see if there are support groups that are available to help you? Have you contacted the Alzheimer's Association to see if they had info on support groups in your area and listed what they offer? These questions are a good start to have you think a little clearer about who to ask and what they do.

Release non-participants

This is a touchy area but is extremely valuable to your peace of mind. What if you come from a big family and let us say, you and your five brother and sisters have all agreed to step in and take care of your mom who has dementia. Mom is a little confused, but still easy to work with. Starting out, it was easy to work with her, but as the disease got worse, mom got a little harder to handle. Mom stopped bathing and refused to change clothes. Mom had a tendency to wander off. Mom developed a foul mouth and berated and insulted everyone that came in her presence. Well, over time, two of your siblings' stress levels got too much to handle. So, they informed you that they had to step away from care to protect their health. You as a primary caregiver could easily take this personally, or you can take the insight you are getting here and know that sometimes, this will happen and one thing to remember is that you cannot let the health of taking care of a loved one diminish the health of your family unit. You have to prayerfully release them from their responsibility and not take it personally. Fight the urge to look at it as a form of deception. Simply know that because you have a plan, you can release them from their roll and still have a functional plan to maintain a quality of care. Overall, your peace of mind and love has to be pushed to its highest level during this process. Letting them go is empowering, and it enables you to release stress. If they came forward and told you, consider it a blessing that they were straightforward with you. That was an honorable thing for them to do and at least they showed you a great deal of respect.

Family dynamic changes

How was your family unit before all this began? Was it an atmosphere of love and respect or was it in turmoil? Was there a spirit of love and respect that existed between you and your loved one? Was your loved one a leader or a supporter? No matter what it was, be prepared for things to change. Change does not have to be bad. But one thing that I am encouraging you to do is to embrace change and master the shift and dynamics of the change. You have to set some emotional goals to achieve for yourself, and you have to take that picture and put it up again the dynamics of the disease. You have to pray and commit that you will hope, pray, and work for maintaining your life goals for your relationship. The disease will present you with many ups and down, but that just means that your life will become a bit more adventurous. Some of the things you experienced may have frightened you, but you have to learn how to manage your response. No matter what you do in life, there will be some troubles you will face, but what matters most is how you choose to respond to what you are experiencing.

Set up family support system and evaluate it bi-weekly

Life, in general, presents a great deal of confusion. If you want to invite confusion into your care plan, one sure fire way is to have too many leaders. In any setting, you will find a wide variety of people. You will have the Type A, direct, analytical person, or you could have the creative, compassionate, free spirit. You could have those that have medical training or those that wish they had medical training and those who would faint at the sight of blood. There are those who can lead and then you have those that follow. With that said, one person has to emerge as the leader and the focal point. My recommendation is this person have the most level head of your bunch. They may not know everything medically or legally, but the person with they have the ability to make an objective decision about how care should be managed. After a leader is selected, that person then needs to identify the other roles and assign key players to each. The leader should let each person know what their role is and thank and encourage them for stepping up and helping out. It is advisable for the leader to have a sit-down review with the team members to make sure they are all on the same page. A good leader will ask questions and dig for observation and feedback. They should be watching for how the team member is handling their role and look for ways to make their roll feel better. They should look for signs of burnout and be prepared and willing to reassign people so not to wear out the team. Trust me when I say, the care could be a long hard road. Some will not have what it takes to go the distance on a fight such as this. You have to face that and, from the depth of your heart of love, be willing to release them from their responsibility without any animosity. Overall, you will want to always add love to the mix. Love for the one you are caring for. Love for your team. Love for yourself. And love for how you are willing to treat everyone involved. Only great things can come from a heart seated in love.

Locate and bring in a geriatric counselor
There are many types of therapists out there. There people who provide counseling for your dog if you so need it and can afford it. There are family councilors, and life and wellness coaches. Along with

this are the emerging groups of councilors that specifically deal with senior adult issues, especially when it comes to any form of mind and brain impairment. If you can get your loved one into one of these sessions, it would prove to be valuable because a skilled counselor can gauge better where your loved one is at emotionally and mentally. Additionally, they can help you manage their stress better and would be able to provide you with insight into things and habits you can implement that could help bring peace and confidence into your loved one's day. Remember, you will want to make sure you, as a caregiver, are listed on the HIPPA form or else the doctor will not be able to work with you in strategizing a plan of care.

Chapter 9 – Dealing with Legal Matters

"A good lawyer knows the law; a great lawyer knows the judge." – Liljay

In this next section, we will talk about some legal considerations. When it comes to legal matters, most people do not usually deal with this until it is too late. This bad timing could cost you more money than you would normally have to spend. It is in your best interest to do some pre-planning. Some of what I am going to present is what you will need to do in reaction to the situations that the disease present, but if you are looking for this guide, I also want you to work on your personal plan for yourself as well as he loved the one you are caring for.

Lawyer and guardian ad litem

For most people, they hardly ever have to deal with an attorney, however, when it comes to probate issues and matters related to an estate, they do come in quite handy and can help you navigate the legal system. If you are going to engage in care for someone, it would be a great idea to find out if they have legal representation. Some people have pre-paid legal service, where they can contact and work with a lawyer, to prepare wills and power-of-attorney forms along with a variety of other legal documents you may need. If they do not have a lawyer, then you can get much of what you need to be processed via probate court, especially if your legal action requires you to set up guardianship. It gets complicated if your loved one is contesting this action. Please remember, they are entitled to legal counsel. So that means they have to have their lawyer involved, or the court will assign a Guardian Ad

Litem (GAL). That is a person who is a court-appointed attorney that represent the rights of infants, unborn, or incompetent individuals in legal matters. In the event of a contested petition before the courts, a GAL will investigate all the facts and review all the laws related to the reason for protest and work with the represented person and petitioner, along with the judge, to come up with a plan that works for the best interest of all. Do not be afraid of or get intimidated by all of this. I have been to court so many times that I feel like I should get a law degree, but I now know how to navigate the legal system to position yourself to provide care and reduce the stress that you may be under while working through all the big issues.

Guardianship

Guardianship is a legal status that enables someone to represent another person who has been declared as being incompetent. That means you can sign documents on their behalf and make most types of decision-related things they would normally have to sign their name to. This comes in handy when signing for bills and certain medical services. It is limited, however, in the event of having to sell declared assets such as cars and homes. It is also limited to certain medical procedures, such as in the event of Do Not Resuscitate (DNR) order. If your loved one has to go to a hospital, the guardianship does no grant you the authorization to execute a DNR order. If that were something you feel you would need, then it would have to be declared to the GAL or lawyer and agreed upon at the time of the guardian request. Also, keep in mind that this order is reviewed annually, and you have to provide a patient update to get your paperwork re-certified. The court order can help save you a lot of hassles. However, it is limited, as I will explain in the next section. The advantage of getting guardian over the power of attorney is that you have court oversight, and it makes it legally clear that there is one focal point of authority when it comes to legal matters. There is more cost involved with this.

What happens after you decide to apply for guardianship?
You should work with your lawyer to:
• Obtain a medical report about the ward from a doctor
• File an application for guardianship with the court
• Serve the proposed ward
• Have an attorney ad litem appointed to represent proposed ward
• Attend a hearing with attorney ad litem and proposed ward
• Obtain a bond
• File an inventory of ward's estate with the court
• File an application for monthly expenditures with the court
• File a plan for management of ward's investments with the court
• File an annual account and report with the court

Conservatorship
   You will want to get conservatorship in the event that your loved one has any significant assets that you will need to manage. It is along the same lines as the guardianship as far as the legal proceedings, and it will give you the needed power to manage a bank account

and retirement funds. You have to keep detailed records of every penny that is spent and the status of all the assets and its assigned value. Many courts require that you make an annual report, and you are to declare at the begging what is the total assets that are in every account. On an annual basis, you will have to give an account of what was spent from each account and the remaining balance has to match the remaining balance of what is in the bank. Both the conservator and guardianship are periodically put under review and are activated based on the re-certification. This stays intact until the event of your loved one passing away. In both the guardianship and the conservatorship, there is a *ward* and a *guardian* or *convocation*. The ward is the person that the judge has declared not to be competent to manage their affairs.

Power of attorney (POA)

A power of attorney (POA) is a private way to decide who will have the legal authority to carry out your wishes if you can no longer speak or act for yourself. It is less costly than a guardianship, which is a public proceeding and the person appointed as your guardian may not be the person you would have chosen. More than likely, to do a power of attorney requires some foreknowledge and planning. That means that if you are the caregiver and power of attorney, your loved one had already anticipated that you are willing and reliable to manage their affairs. With the POA, you can divide the power up among different people. Some of the ways I have seen it divided is POA for Healthcare, POA for Financial, and Durable POA. In this case, the person who you are caring for has designated and wanted this level of support. The Durable POA gives a person power to make decisions even in the event of incapacitation.

With a POA, there is the *principal* and the *agent*. The principal is the person making the request, and the agent is the person that will carry out the wishes.

The advantage of the POA over the guardianship is that it keeps the principal in charge while granting someone (the agent) to act on his or her behalf. Bear in mind that some banks exercise the right not to honor the POA, whereas the conservatorship gives you the authority of the court system to conduct banking on their behalf.

Last will, living trust, and living will

Above, we looked at how things are managed while the loved one is living, in this next section, we will look at how to asset management in the event of their passing. I am no expert in this area, but if you have any assets to manage or placed in charge of managing, here are some things to consider. All of the following explanations of wills and trusts come from *LegalZoom.com*. The last will is used to distribute property to beneficiaries, specify last wishes, and name guardians for minor children. It is an important part of any estate plan. Without one, the courts will make these critical decisions for you.

A will is a legal document that directs the disposition of your assets after your death. Having a valid will makes the probate process and the distribution of your assets, go more smoothly than if you did not have a will. Also, in a will, you can name a guardian for your children.

A living trust is used to transfer property to beneficiaries. But, unlike the last will, a living trust is not usually subject to probate court, which can take years and cost thousands in attorney and court fees. A living trust is a legal document that becomes valid when you execute the documents and transfer property. Your loved one, as the grantor and trustee, manage the assets while they are alive, and then they are passed directly to a trustee of their choice upon their death without involving probate.   Although you cannot name a guardian for your children in a living trust, you can, however, choose someone to manage assets set aside for a specific beneficiary until they are older. As discussed below, you can execute a will in conjunction with your living trust, under which you can name a guardian of your children. Moreover, a living trust helps you avoid the cost and delays of probate, it keeps the details of your estate private, and it may reduce certain estate taxes.

A living will lets you outline important healthcare decisions in advance, such as whether or not to remain on artificial life support. It also can help makes decisions about life support and specify organ donation in the event that your loved on passes away.

The main difference between a will and a living trust is that a will takes effect only after your death while a living trust becomes valid as soon as it is duly executed and assets are added—that is, during your lifetime. Another significant difference between the two is that a living trust can make provisions for your estate in case you are incapacitated. A will cannot do this, although a power of attorney can. Living trusts, though, may be more specific and make managing the estate easier on the trustee than a power of attorney. Moreover, regarding probate, a living trust can help to avoid time and costs associated with it, particularly because with a living trust, there is no freezing of assets so long as there's a funded trust. Another advantage of a living trust is that it remains private in many states while a will becomes part of the public record during the probate process.

What factors should I consider when choosing between a living trust and a will?

Some of the most important factors to consider when deciding on whether you should establish a living trust include, but are not limited to, the following:

1. Your location- state law regarding estate taxes and probate vary greatly, so what may be advantageous in one state may not be in another.

2. Your assets- states establish an asset value below which even wills can bypass probate, but that does not mean lower valued estates could not benefit from the other advantages of a living trust. Also, if you have assets that could be harmed by prolonged probate, such as a business, for example, a living trust might be the better choice.

3. Taxes- s living trust may have estate tax advantages both on the federal and state levels, but it depends not only on your state and the value of your estate, but also on the federal estate tax, the status of which is currently in limbo.

4. Your beneficiaries- because a living trust can hold your assets after your death, it offers a way to provide for young, special needs, or other particular beneficiaries you would rather not immediately receive their share of your estate. You may also provide for the care of pets in this way.

5. The likelihood of a contested estate- if you think there is a good chance of this happening, a living trust may be more likely to withstand the challenge.

6. Your trust in a potential trustee- with a living trust, you must be able to trust your named trustee to act according to your wishes without court intervention or monitoring.

7. Your current financial situation- setting up a living trust may be more expensive upfront than writing a will, but this must also be weighed against all the above factors.

Final thoughts on a living trust

With a living trust, an asset does not become part of it without specifically being included, so you must keep up with adding your assets to the trust to ensure that a valued asset does not end up going through probate, especially if it is not included in your will either. For this reason, it is also advisable to have a pour-over will, not only because you can name a guardian for any children, but also because you can catch any assets that did not make it into the trust. Like all wills, a pour-over will is handled in probate court if necessary.

Chapter 10 - Lifestyle Dynamics

"Courage doesn't always roar. Sometimes courage is the quiet voice at the end of the day saying 'I will try again tomorrow,'" – Unknown

In this section, I am going to share with you some secrets that I learned along the way. Dementia took me to a whole new level as a person and liberated my thinking and conduct. It helped me address some things on an emotional level that solidified my outlook on my identity, my relationship with my sister, the level of care I realistically provide and mostly, how I was choosing to care for myself. In the next few sections, I will get into the heart of the relationship I had with my sister and the impact she had on me, as well as the impact the disease took on our way of life.

What do you still like about them?

"The deeper your scars, the more room there is to fill them up with love. Don't hate your scars, appreciate their depth." – Daniel Chidiac

When I was first personally introduced to this disease, my heart was not in a good place. I was angry and bitter. I was off balance and tried to make heads or tails of everything. God, why? How could you let this disease hit our family like this? As hard as we worked and served him and his kingdom, it was shocking to have something like this happen. The disease made my sister bitter and presented her in a hateful manner.

After a period of dealing with this disease, I had to come in contact with some great council. A question arose from one of our talks that was so profound, it stuck with me even now: "what is it you still like your loved one?" That question was pointed and challenging.

As mad as I was, did I still love my sister and did I still like her? Even though, at the time, my sister did not have a memory of her own of how thing were between us, I still did. I own them and in spite of the circumstance, I cherished them. I remembered how she cared for me and when there were big events in my life, no matter even if we were odds, she still supported me with love. Just like any siblings, we had our rivalries, but we also had our love. That question caused me to find the energy, passion, and purpose to hang in there and find a better way to deal with the frustration that this disease could cause. Love was and still is the core of my heart, and love had to be the key to usher in freedom and liberty into the care I needed to give to my sister.

Release what you had for a stronger today
"God doesn't give us what we can handle; He helps us handle what we have been given." – Unknown

A person's vantage point can determine how they remember their past—either positively or negatively. My sister and I fought like cats and dogs. There were times I despised her when I was a young child because she spanked me like my mother would when I got out of line. As I got older from my adolescent, I developed more respect for my sister and she became one of my biggest supporters. I remember how happy I was when my I got to see my sister at family gatherings. Now, do not get me wrong. I may have been happy to see her, but in no way, was I going to let her know that. I gave her the hardest time possible. I would talk to her in a way to get her dialed up. But we both knew it was done out of love.

As fond as those memories were, it was hard to see her after the disease did its damage on her. I was longing for and missing the times of earlier years. When I saw her, there was a normal body that seemed healthy, but when she spoke, it was painfully obvious that she was not the same person I grew up with. I was angry because I felt a deep loss. I wanted to hold on to what she was. I wanted her to engage in the things she uses to do. It pained me to watch her eat. She lost all dexterity and coordination.

I had to come to grips with the pain I was experiencing. I wanted to hang on so badly to what it used to be, and not open my eyes to what my reality actually was. I had to pray, work, and understand that I could not go back to the way our lives once were. Each day, a person helping someone with dementia requires a growing strength. Not just physical strength, but the spiritual strength to give you vision and insight as to how to handle yourself inside of the chaos that is going around you. You have to have insight so you can have the means to shine brightly and dispel the darkness.

Release the f-words (flexibility and forgiveness)
"Stay committed to your decision, but stay flexible in your approach." – Tony Robbins

As you address the needs of a person with dementia, I have heard and personally witnessed the use of the F-bomb. When my sister got agitated, and felt threatened, she would do her best to defend herself. Most of what was getting her dialed up was things that were made up in here mind. So she would lash out at anyone and everyone. She would let words I did not even think she knew.   She had no control of her expression, and I knew it was not her that was tearing into me.

As she grew to express herself in demonstrative ways, I had to counter that with alternative F-Words. I had to learn to respond with a great deal of flexibility. I had to become more flexible in my agenda and my presentation to her. I had to relearn her new likes and dislikes and become gentler in my expression. Now, that was hard for me to learn. I am a very schedule oriented individual. It is core to my military training. The clock managed everything, and there was no place for emotions or sentiments. However, I found a new source of power in being flexible. By choosing to slow things down, it forced me to take more in and examine things in my life that I enjoyed, and it allowed me to ask the question: "why?" I now regularly ask why I did the things I do. I ask what is the result that I want to accomplish, beyond just saying that I got something done. I had to become observant and determined to find meaning and purpose in my activity. By becoming more flexible, I was equipped and enabled with tools to defuse quickly stress that existed in my day.

The other F-word I had to practice was forgiveness. I need to be clear and deliberate about forgiving my sister for getting this disease. It was not her fault, and there was nothing she did to trigger this disease. I had to forgive even, anybody or anything that I suspected of contributing to here disease. By blaming others, I was eroding my mental support and power to have a joyful relationship with my sister. I had to forgive myself for being angry and lashing out at my sister when she was clearly having difficulties with processing her thoughts. I had to forgive others that agreed to help me care for my sister, but over time, bailed on me and left me holding the bag. Above all, I had to forgive God for allowing all of this to happen. If I kept hanging on to that pain and frustration, it would have slowly killed me physically and above all, spiritually. I give thanks to God for sending the right people to come along side me and to help me with my feelings and help me with my care of my sister. Forgiveness has brought me so much liberty.

Do not make judgment calls

***"You never really understand a person until you consider things from his point of view … Until you climb into his skin and walk around in it." – Harper Lee,* To Kill and Mockingbird**

Who am I to judge? What do I have to judge about? Do I find myself being judgmental about my loved one or members of my support team? Is it fair to judge and if so, am I fair because I am choosing to judge? These are some great questions that many people do not take the time to address. One other question is, what is all the judging doing to my life and spirit? Is it causing my heart to function from a weakened state?

It is my passion that you feel inspired and have hope as you stand up to provide care. Some of you may be going gung-ho and going all out on your level of care and others are lost in the tall grass. No matter where you are, you are going to be all right. Take a moment to stop. Take a deep breath and look around. There is hope, and there is freedom. But I must warn you, by proceeding with a critical, judgmental spirit, you will become debilitated in your ability to love and to serve. So, take the time to be honest with yourself and those around you. Be real and clear in your knowledge and your situation. Judge with the same measure you would want granted to you.

Know your life and show up for it
"The tragedy in life doesn't lie in not reaching your goals. The tragedy lies in having no goals to reach." – Benjamin E. Mays

I am expressing this as a warning that was imparted to me a while ago. When things are going a mile a minute, and you are getting tossed about and feel ripped from the inside out, this is the time you have to put on the mental breaks. First of all, ask yourself, who were you before all of this began? What did you do for a career? Who were you connected with? What were you passionate about and how did you show it? You may feel resentment toward the life you life right now because you feel like this disease robbed you of something valuable. But to look at it that way means that you are willing to ingest mental poison.

My heartfelt advice is to be real, clear and deliberate with yourself as a caregiver. Your life has taken on a role as caregiver, but do not fall into the trap of treating it like a prison. Your life beyond the care you provide matters. Do not fool yourself and take on a false send of nobility by giving your all to your loved one. I am pleading with you to find some balance to engage in things that still allow for you to be you. You were given and granted skills and talent for a reason. Do not allow yourself to kill that uniqueness that God has birthed inside you.

Every day, in every way, be deliberate to show up for your life. If you like to sew, take a few minutes every day to practice your skills. If your passion is speaking, if you cannot get out of your crowd, you can at least record your expressions and release your topics online. But either way, you *must* fight for your life and identify. Never let that die or go down because you chose to love and help out.

You cannot go back, but you can be real and go forward

"Every day we have a choice. We can live in fear or move forward in faith." – Billy Cox

It is normal to sit and reflect on the pleasant memories of yesterday. There is no real harm in that on the surface. However, there are some hidden traps that could send you down an emotional rabbit trail that you may seriously struggle to return from. You have to ask yourself, how much time are you spending looking back and then do you have a purpose or a compelling reason for you to be looking back so much. When we look back, we commonly find a place and time where we felt joy and empowerment. There were events that took us on a euphoric high. This memory took us to a place that we felt confident. As great as those memories were, we have to be mindful not to get caught up in trying to recreate those events. It took a great deal of random and calculated events to bring together the memories you cherished and to try to recreate that, would take a miracle from God.

When you stepped up to take care of your loved one, it took heart and courage to move into the position of caregiver. And what a noble and valiant person you are. You enlisted in a war that was not your own, but you chose to serve and battle the darkness. Like a good soldier, you cannot, in the heat of batter, take inventory of your loss. You have to assess what you have and focus on the mission at hand. You have to be real about your role, the tools you have, and your skills to use them. Then you must stand up, press on, and move forward.

I am not expressing that I want you to get fired up and drive so fast and hard that you mow over your loved one, but what I am deeply expressing is that you need to be clear on where you are headed and how you want to get there. Take a deep assessment of not how much you are willing to sacrifice, but ask yourself if the sacrifice is worth it and balance what you are giving up as you press ahead in the level of care you are willing to commit.

Your attitude sets the pace
"The greatest discovery in any generation is that a human being can alter his life by altering his attitude."
– William James

Most people want to have a good day. We want to have nice weather. We want to have great friends and family to connect with. We want to have peace in our day. However, most of us know that life is not wired that way, where everything works out smooth and perfect. We are going to have storm clouds and wind. We are going to get some rain on our parades. Life has a lot of twists and turns that can take you on a journey that could suck the life right out of you. That is a given. But we all have been granted a tool and power to navigate and overcome the obstacles life puts in our way. We may not be granted the means to move the obstacle or resolve the present problem, but one thing we have absolute power over and that is our view and interpretation of how we are looking at the situation.

My sister would make me so angry because I was a person on a tight schedule. My work was demanding, and my sister caused a lot of problems on my job and things that I needed to do with my day. There were times where I would let my frustrations show. And I would let my attitude get the best of me. There was a time my sister and I got into shouting matches because we had similar attitudes. Neither of us was the type that would back down from a fight. There were times before and after the disease was diagnosed that we would have face-to-face shouting matches because neither of us would give.

I am so grateful that I got help from friends that could speak to my spirit and let me know, in spite of the disease, my attitude was the rudder of my life that determines if I was going to be in peace or troubled waters. My attitude determined the peace and pace of my life. I had to fight to get that under control. I had to stay continuously aware of how my attitude influenced the environment and other attitudes around me. I had to take full ownership of that, and I had to convert my attitude from being a baseball bat and make it into a catcher's mitt. There were days where my sister would blast me because she felt uncomfortable. I had to learn how to absorb that energy and redirect it so that it would produce the highest possible outcome for the given situation. Now, this does not negate that there were some out of control moments, but I was armed with wisdom and knowledge that I had the power to shorten the storms and take away some of its intensity but simply adjusting my attitude.

Be a victor and not a victim

"Focus on the positive, defend your mind against the negative, and expect victory." – Billy Cox

It is easy to cry foul on the play of life and to throw in the towel. We join in the chorus of "woe is me." We can roll on the floor and cry like a baby and say life is not fair. Now, I do not want to minimize your feeling but the truth is hard to deal with, and the reality is, life is not supposed to be fair. Life is full of hits, twist, and turns. Life has things that will hurt, kill, and maim you. However, God has granted mankind with the ability to adapt and overcome. By stopping and taking deep account of your pain and failure, it could easily but you into the victim spirit of influence. As you start to complain and blame, you also start to collect other complainers in your life. Let me restate, this book is about helping you, as a caregiver, develop a healthy and strong lifestyle and being a victim does not resemble that of being healthy. I am introducing a dream shift and encouraging you to be deliberate of changing your metaphorical view on your life. The reality is that things are tough, but by faith and correct action based on sound knowledge, you can adjust the odds of your life. You can overcome and make a huge difference in your environment and through sound action, you can enhance your faith in what will be. Stay determined and focused, and stay in the fight and do not let the pain overshadow your hope.

Dis-ease causes disease

"Your difficulty, your disease, your conflicts are preparing you to be a voice of encouragement to your brothers." – Max Lucado

What you are facing as a caregiver will not be easy by any stretch of the imagination. For most, this disease brings out the worst in a loved one. There is a lot of physical and emotional strain that develops as a result. That strain can cause all sorts of problems in you that may impact you inside and out. It a proven fact that a person under a great deal of stress can develop hypertension. When we are stressed, we also like to reach for the high in sugar and fatty comfort foods that will help us pack on pounds. Along with the pounds come arterial blockage, which is essentially high cholesterol. Too much stress can impact how the brain functions and could impact your mental health.

To combat these symptoms, it would be a great idea to see your physician, but another thing I would prescribe for you to plan at least one day a week of quiet time for yourself. You need to wind down to prevent a meltdown. Go to the spa. Get your mani pedi. Go to the park and take in some sunshine. Take time to relax and breathe.

The temptation is to guilt yourself into back-breaking, copious service and treat your care as a form of punishment. However, what this will lead to, for some, is an early demise and a load of stress a caregiver will have, especially if you have not set up a care plan that should kick-in in the event of your untimely demise. So, consider being deliberate and taking time out and try to practice taking it easy.

Thought affirmations

"People often say that motivation doesn't last. Well, neither does bathing. That is why we recommend it daily." – Zig Ziglar

In our cynical society, we are conditioned to practice and use thought destroying metaphors to describe our life situations. Such as, if you are having difficulties with your kids, many would say, "I'm a bad parent." If we make a mistake at work, we may say, "I'm an idiot." When it comes to caring for our loved ones, we could get hung up on having a "miserable day." Our loved one could have had a recent fit of rage or simply refused to cooperate. They may have wondered off, or you had a rough experience with trying to get them to bathe. With these difficulties, it is easy to feel broken and defeated if you choose to take it personally. My hope with this is to heighten your awareness and help you to release yourself from the problem. You are not the problem. Your interaction with your loved one is not the problem. But a huge part of the problem is how you choose to view yourself and the situation you are under. What you think about yourself matters when it comes to what you can and will do. A practice I use is arresting my thoughts. I have alarms set on my phone that goes off every 2 hours. The alarms are my reminder to examine the types of thoughts I have been thinking lately. If they are of a negative nature, I demand myself to dig in and figure out why I am on a cycle of destructive thinking. If there is no real and solid reason, then I command myself to stopping the negative thinking dead in its tracks. Next, within that same setting, I make myself obligated to think of something good about myself, what I am doing, and even about the person that I am caring for. I have to stay focused and committed to owning the thoughts that I allow to invade my brain. I do not give myself room or permission to engage with stray thoughts. I push myself to take my thoughts to a higher level with the goal of getting the best out of life.

A part of living with the disease is living
"Live the life you love. Love the life you live." – Bob Marley

There is no real or solid cure for this disease at this time. We know that inevitably, our loved one dies. It hurts to face that fact. We still hold out in hope. We pray and fight for them to get better. We lay it on the line, and we even take on guilt for what our loved one is experiencing. It hurts to see them this way. Some of us cry daily as we stay in the fight and give our all in care. We fight until death. Some have come to the conclusion that if our loved one is dying, then we choose to let the best part of our hearts die along with them. We take on limiting beliefs that encourage us to be martyrs.

But, if you are reading this book and have made it this far, you must have held on to the fact that your life is valuable and has a higher meaning. You have come to the realization that what you are going through at the moment is not the sum of your life. It is just a small piece, compared to the bigger scheme of life. Your life has value. You are not alone and are not the first person in history to go through what you are facing. There is hope, and you have to be determined to not let you care suck the life right out of you. Make it a point to check in on your life. Examine the whole health of your life.

If you are not putting deliberate actions into promoting signs of life onto your day, then by default you are inviting death.   I am not saying neglect your responsibility for care, but what I am saying is take moments to reflect, refresh, and recharge. You owe it to yourself, as well as your loved one.

Adjusting to the new normal
"If you are always trying to be normal, you will never know how amazing you can be." – Maya Angelou

For some, you used to have a routine where you got up every morning, stretched and worked out. Showered and got ready for work. Worked a full day and made a difference on your job and then came home to have your family greet you and then spend quality time with them till it was time to go to bed and start the cycle all over again. Others traveled for living or pleasure while others are artists who spend their day singing, painting, dancing or in another kind of way they chose to give their expression.

Today, the schedule looks a little different. You rise in the morning ahead of everyone. You then check in on your loved one and ask them if they want breakfast for that day. You may even have to check their vitals if you are trained in that area. Your day could be loaded with cooking, cleaning, and changing clothes multiple times in a day. Running errands along with transporting. You may even have to do direct feedings, catheter replacement, bathing, and changing of adult garments. You have a full day.

There may be a huge contrast from what you use to do, versus what you are doing today or may soon be engaging in.   No matter what, it will require some adjustment. For some, it does not take much to make that transition, but for others, there could be total and downright resistance.

I can say for certain; it was hard for me to make my changes. I am a business owner. I am a mover and shaker, and it was hard for me to be tied down with the responsibility that went with providing care. I did not know what to give up from my life for this. What changed for me was being able to see the bigger picture. Everything that I was going for in business, I was achieving in the level of care I was providing to my sister. I wanted to be respected and empowered. My sister gave me respect in the best way she could with her limited capacity. I was empowered by my sister and granted authority by the circuit court to govern over and protect the life of my sister. I had to inherit my reason for caring to make the transition. Deep down inside, I loved my sister. I felt pity for her when I witnessed how she tried to navigate life and struggled at it. What was once work turned into a blessing for both of us. I experienced tremendous growth and clarity when it came to my interaction with her as well as with other people. My level of care helped me to become more gracious and appreciative of life and more willing to incorporate the help of others. The level of care I provided taught me how to be a better listener and to listen with my ears and eyes and let it touch my heart before I tried to interpret what was being said. Simply said, you have to open your heart and give a little on your agenda to experience peace and personal growth through this endeavor.

Be real and clear with what your goals are and know that it is all right to change

"Change your thoughts and you change the word." – Norman Vincent Peale

It is normal to want to set goals. It is pounded into us as a key to achieving any success. We are encouraged to write our goals down and plan when we will reach them. We are taught to burn with passion until we reach said goal. Nothing is wrong with any of that thinking. We should have clear and attainable goals. However, we must understand the shifting and contrasting difference in our mind and the minds of our loved ones when it comes to goals. The value of agendas and goals diminishes to a person dealing with dementia. Goals and agendas become the enemy. Time loses its importance to them because the part of brain that tracks time deteriorates. To them, agenda become a threat.

Once again, it is all right to have goals, but as a caregiver you have to do an assessment of the goals that you have and come to the conclusion that some goals may have to be put off for a season, or you may have to lighten the agenda so not to cause stress for your home environment. Give yourself the power and freedom to master, change and adjust what comes into and out of your life and decide for health sake what will manage your time.

There are some cut and dry events that happen in your day that you cannot change, and there are others that if you did not do it, it might be inconvenient for you or someone else, but life could still go on even if you did not participate. You have to know what your goals are when it comes to caregiving and your personal life, business life, and you have to think, pray, meditate, and reason to find a balance and workflow that is healthy for you. If taking care of your loved one is completely halting your personal life goals, then you must make the clear and conscious decision to get qualified help. There is no shame in asking for help. There is only regret if you choose not to.

The power of the presence of the moment
"Realize deeply that the present moment is all you ever have." – Eckhart Tolle

A very powerful tool that you should think about adding to your arsenal is the power of presence. What this simply means is being attentive to the moment you are in and observing every element of that moment. Not just time and how much you can fit into that moment, but allowing yourself to utilize your five senses and all these sensations to speak to your emotions.

Most people are short and insensitive with others in such a way that they have a lot of difficulties communicating. By being present, you are engaging at full mind, body, and spirit level to the person that you are interacting with. Being present causes you to communicate at an empathetic level. You do not just hear the words your loved one is saying, but you are connecting to such a heightened emotional state that helps you look at not what is being communicated, but why.

When a person with dementia communicates, there are gaps that exist and by you choosing to be really in tune with them, you are granted a deeper mastery over expressions. You can learn to ask the right questions in the right way and patiently listen. This also shows a high level of respect for your loved one and in turn creates an environment where they feel safe, respected, and confident. It reduces aggression and stress that may arise in a given communication dilemma. Exercising presence grants you a means to overcome a great deal of emotion and communication obstacles.

Release the life you had to find and see the benefit of today.
"Quit beating you up. You are not a finished a product. You are still a work in progress." – Joel Osteen

"I gave up my life for all of this. It hurts so bad to see my dad in this way, and I want to do all that I can to make his life better. But I can't help but be angry because I had to give up my promising career so that I can take time out to give all of this care for him. I felt like life ripped me off." These deep expressions are what many are going through as they try to sort out what happened to their life. It seems like an unfair exchange. For many, this digs up strong emotions and can come across as deep-seated resentment for those that we care about. It seems as if we are forced to give up everything we ever fought for. Why? Is it all worth it? Those are some big questions. They can only be addressed by the sentiment of the person we want to become and how we choose to let the situation shape us. Trust me when I say, it is easy to get bitter and very hard to find a way to get better, especially, if we choose to go it alone. We can convince ourselves to take the victim mentality.

So, what are we holding on to and by choosing not to care for our loved one for a season, are we letting go? I am challenging you to consider what you had and then to consider how not to let it go, but to temporarily set it aside while you assess what you are doing and why. I am also asking what type of care you want to provide and assess what you hope to gain from your relationship as you provide your love and care.

Trust me when I say it is not a bad thing to let go. The letting go is where you can gain a greater perspective on what is really important. Sometimes things and activity are not as important as we have allowed ourselves to be convinced. There are benefits and beauty in the everyday and every situation if we are diligent and willing to seek it. But that can only come when we chose to get to a peaceful place in our heart. If we are passionate about controlling life too much, we will never find the means to be at pace.

Never say never

"Never say never, because limits, like fear, are often just an illusion." – Michael Jordan

I believe and support the idea of setting and maintaining standards. Many great things would never have been invented if it were not for high standards. Standards describe the height and depth of what is possible. Standards help us to know what we can say "yes" to and what we should say "no" to. Standards drive who we let into our lives and who we should consider stepping away from. However, we must put a distinguishing factor between what we are doing and why. It is easy to get caught up in "the what" at the expense of "the why".

Let me be frank. To care for someone requires a deep, heartfelt commitment. It has a lot of twists and turns in it. It is a dim road that many shy away from. If you have a deep connection to the person you are caring for, then it becomes extremely hard to see what they are going through. If you are caring for them early in the game, then know what I am going to reveal could shock you to the point to making you walk away.

I want to challenge you not only to set high standards, but I also want you to look at why you have set them and to know when to shift them for the righter purpose. Clearly measure your life goals against a fixed foundation. If your goal is to work your way up the corporate ladder, ask why? What type of person were you hoping to become once you achieved that goal? What meaning have you fixed to that goal? What value was that goal supposed to bring to your life?

I am not saying give up on your life goals and jump in with all your being to become a caregiver. No one in their right mind would want to do this, but I can say, by engaging in doing this, you can adjust a more noble reason on what this means to you. It does take commitment and sacrifice to serve. It takes heart and a higher caliber of thinking. But, by no mean should you let yourself feel bad for adjusting to caring. Do not falsely think of yourself as a quitter because you chose to care for someone and to put your career aside. There are greater rewards in store for you for taking this leap of faith.

You will sweat, cry, and bleed in this arena. You will get frustrated. You will feel pain. You may never hear the words "thank you." But you can, and you will, change lives beyond measure based on the level of care you choose to step up too.

Four out of five families fall apart as a result of caring for someone with dementia

"Coming together is a beginning, staying together is progress, and working together is success." – Henry Ford

My family is big, by my standard. My mother had 13 siblings. I have seven siblings. I have 26 nephews and nieces. I have a large number of great nephews and nieces. I have a ton of cousins and loved ones in the area. I can remember a time when we would have some seriously large family gathering that would rival to none. We were a loving and supportive family. However, when you have a loved one that is going through something as ugly as dementia, things change. It is a horrible disease that strips away from the heart and character of someone who was once lovable.

If you want to break a strong family, let someone who is strong have to care for someone who is sick with a catastrophic illness. I saw so much of my family drift away when they started to realize how hard it would be to care for my sister. In her last three years of her life, she required round the clock care. There was a lot of sleep lost and a lot of time spent. Some families are lovable and close, but when faced with this, they lose sight and hope. On average, four out of every five families fall apart as a result of long-term care. What I mean by fall apart is where there were closeness and support, is now distance and desertions. There were fingers of accusation of who was caring better than the next, or who was neglecting more than the other. Fights develop about who is going to pay for everything. Discussions come up about where the loved one will live and be cared for. Battles come up about if they are cared for at home or in an assisted living facility or nursing home. Fights break out over accepting if your loved one requires hospice care or not.

I am giving you this information so you can be aware, or to confirm what you may be currently walking through. If you are aware of what may happen, you can then choose how you will either face it or what you can do about it. We talked earlier about how to build a strong, varied team. If you can do this, then it can take off some of the strain of your family as you move forward with care and it can give you the right frame of mind to know when to release people from their responsibility without having animosity. In the end, you do not want to walk away with a crush or bruised heart simply because people chose to be real and admit that they could not handle what was in front of them. It is good to release in love.

Do not ever lie and promise you will never send them to a nursing home
"Honesty does not always bring a response of love, but it is essential to it." – Ray Blanton

It is a hard vision for many caregivers to decide when a person should go into nursing care. Many feel like they have failed their loved one and like they are giving up. They treat such a move as a failure. In my case, I had no intention of putting my sister in a home. When I saw here, I saw a proud woman. Dementia had made her rough around the edges and difficult to get along with, but she was still my sister, and she asked me to take care of her. I risked it all to take care of her. I put my family, my job, and finances at risk while caring for her. It hurt when I saw the seizures come, and when she was on the ground shaking and I had no clue what to do. I know full well I was out of depth. I knew a decision had to be made. But I also felt like I was betraying her by putting her in a nursing home.

When I got her started in adult day care, she was so angry that she had to go to a new place to be locked in a room and not be allowed to walk the streets. I felt bad that I was taking her freedom from her, but I knew she was in danger because she was getting lost and there were times she would leave and I would be caught with searching high and low trying to locate her. That was a scary and sinking feeling.

But I know that as hard as it is to make the decision to place them in a home, it is harder to have promised you would never place them there then to later go back on your word. That will become heartbreaking to them if they are consciously aware of what is taking place.   I would advise you to use every form of diversion not to make that promise. If they press the matter, you will have to tell them in a clear and diplomatic manner.   This conversation might look something like this: "I would love to have you stay with me forever. I know it gets hard at times, but I promise to make sure you get the best care possible, no matter where we are." By saying this you are not promising to keep them out of a home, but you are committing to care for them in every way possible. So, be truthful, but stay tactful. Tact will reduce stress and prolong cognitive function in their life. You are giving them hope, but not false hope.   Practice honesty and tenderhearted expression.

You may need to let go of what was, and move to what is

"Don't let the sadness of your past and the fear of your future ruin the happiness of your present!" – **Unknown**

My sister used to have a fashion line. She would develop her clothing line and promote her fashion shows. She also made her jewelry. She was ambitious about her career and wealth. She was busy and active in the pursuit of who she was. She loved to live life without limits. She inspired me to do the same. That made dealing with this disease so much more devastating.

When I started caring for her, I was determined to find the best way to care for her and to find a cure. I read and asked questions. I researched everything that came my way. I wanted her well. I prayed and envisioned her well. I had people pray for her. I believed she could get her life back. Through all that effort, I saw so much failure. My heart broke over watching her in pain. I felt like a quitter because I could not find the help she needed. This is not right. This is not fair. Why, dear God, would you let such a disease touch a loving person in this way?

With all the grief I was going through, I had to adjust and grow by knowing what I could change and work on. I also grew by knowing what I had to accept and let go of. I had to move out of what was and learn to maximize every moment of every day. By doing such, I was enabled to receive liberty, peace, and hope.

"Take me home"

"Sometimes you will never know the true value of a moment until it becomes a memory." – Unknown

"Take me home, I want to go home! I want to go home now!" When you hear this, you have reached a moment of frustration that is very difficult to address. It may seem simple to try to solve. You could be out at an event, and your loved one may experience a situation that creates some form of anxiety and they may demand to go home. But you have to understand that a person with dementia is experiencing their foundation and stability slowing being stripped away. So, home may not be a place where they live, but a representation of what they remember where they felt safe and secure. Home could be their childhood home. Home could be a blanket that they felt comfortable under. Home could be taking a look at a clear blue sky. Bottom line, "home" is code for they are looking for a calmer setting so they can feel secure.

It is important to get to know them and to try to get a good composite of their life. If you can start working with them early in the disease, you should try to ask as many questions as you can about their life, and try to record it and from those memories you can identify what they consider vital and key to their existence.

In my sister's case, when she would get some place that was new, like a busy store, or a concert, or even church, she would get overwhelmed by the crowds. The lights and noise would raise her stress level. The tension would cause her to lash out with strong expressions. She would get so angry and would want to go home. There were times where certain events turned into disaster. What I wish I knew early on was how people impaired by dementia processed various stimuli.

She felt insecure with all the changes that were going on. She would say, "I want to go home." And there were times I left certain events and took her home, but she would still be agitated and say that it was not her home. I got confused by what she was saying and not working to find out what she was meaning. Verbal communication is not an exact science or means of expression with dementia. "Home" to her meant a place, event or object where she felt safe, secure and in charge. In her case, she had pictures that she would carry around that she would like to look at to help anchor her memory. To get her to calm down at times, I would place the picture of our family in her hands. She got to see people she still knew and smiled on their faces, and this would bring in a strong sense of peace. You need to find what calms your loved one and be armed and ready to present it when thing flair up.

Be aware of momentary performance
"The greatest deception men suffer is from their opinion." -Leonardo Da Vinci
This was a confusing issue I had to address when caring for my sister. She had momentary lapses of cognitive skills that she could pull together early on in the disease that she would use to mask and confuse doctors about how she was doing. When I would take her to the doctor or to places where she would meet someone new for the first time, she would go into this act that made her seem like she was not dealing with a

disease, and would totally confuse me about where she was with the disease.

During an examination, it was totally baffling how her personality would switch when we got in the presence of the doctor. She would take on a false sweet demeanor in her interaction. However, there were some tell-tell signs that there were issues, because of how she would respond. She would answer though questions on memory issues with short, harsh responses and with a slight angry attitude. But overall, she did her best to maintain her performance, until we left the office. My advice to you is to be aware of this and to exercise patience. Observe how they function and anticipate the change so you can better respond and address any issues that may pop up.

Be aware of visual issues and the new center of gravity
"The best and most beautiful things in the world cannot be seen or even touched – they must be felt with the heart." -Helen Keller

As I said earlier, there are changes that hit most patients due to changes in the brain. They may go from 20/20 to binocular vision where they lose their peripheral vision. Their vision could then shift to monocular vision, where they get a direct, in front, head on focus, and it will cause them to lose depth perception. This will greatly impact how they move and how they stand. If an object is not right in front of them and their sight, then that object does not exist. That means that if they in your home, and you are taking care of them, it would be best to arrange the furniture and sturdy objects so that they are at the right height and that you intentionally create narrow walkways so they can have things to grab onto as they traverse your living environment. This methodology is better than having them use a walker. Because they have a lower and forward center of gravity, as well as visual impairments and muscular complication, they are prone to fall over the walker, not to mention, they may forget they require a walker to get around. A walker could be used when going to places other than home, but it would be better in the home to adjust the furniture layout to grant them stability and confidence.

You can have a short visit that goes well vs. an hour that goes right
"Life isn't a matter of milestone, but of moments." – Rose Kennedy

I have seen some caregivers who try to swing for the fences when it comes to interaction with their loved ones. This is a difficult concept to come to terms with, but we must all understand, that every day will not be the same and the points of connections that were there yesterday, will not be there tomorrow. Consider yourself blessed if you got to care for your loved one during the early stages of the disease. In this phase, you may have been able to do and enjoy things with them. But as parts of them and their identity slips away, you may feel frustration as to why you cannot have a simple conversation with your mom or grandma. You will try acts of kindness and in response, you will get rough and abrasive answers. You will experience short tempers and moments of rage as you move into the mid to later stages of the disease.

But, there is something to look forward to as long as you can adjust your level of expectation. First, understand that they cannot help it. You cannot make them understand how rude they are being. The rational center of their brain is slowly deteriorating. So allow me to set a new standard. Aim for short moments of good times sandwiched within the frustration and rage. You may not be able to adjust what they are throwing at you, but you get to choose how you are going to receive it. I pray you can stay above the mess, and rise to a higher plain. Adjust yourself so that your peace comes from within and not from what you are experiencing externally. I have learned to live by the rule that happiness does not come from what I experience. My happiness is what I choose to manufacture and project. If I let happiness come from my external, then I have no choice over how I feel. But if I dwell on what makes me happy, and act on it, then I have better control of the circumstances.

Activities matter

Was your loved one a dancer, a singer, or an artist? Did they love nature, swimming, or where they into sports? It would be very therapeutic for you to find a way to help them do the things they used to love again, and it may even be helpful for you to join them in any capacity that you can. By doing this, you will have a strong connection point with who they were and when times are rough, you will have a connection point to talk with them about, to reinforce their memory. You will find that as time goes on, the more you talk to them about their memories and observe and write what you experience, you will have not only something to help them remember but something special to remember them by. You will also want to persuade them to simplify their activities and put it at a level that they are challenged, but not overwhelmed. If they have to struggle too much with old activities they used to love, they will get frustrated and embarrassed and decide to give up because they will not want to have another thing that they feel they have failed.

Chapter 11 - Time Management

"The key is not to prioritize what you schedule, but to schedule your priority." – Steven Covey

There are some important features you will want to master when it comes to time management that is unlike what you have been taught. Traditional time management tends to push and drive toward a goal, but when it comes to time management with a person with dementia, it becomes persuasion and channeling focus. I will reveal what I mean within this section.

Daily activity plan

"Happy people plan actions, they don't plan results." – Denis Waitley

Take a good look at how your day is structured and what you are choosing to pack into your personal day. Do you have every waking hour loaded with activity? How much downtime is planned into your schedule? For a normal person with no mental impairment, a busy schedule could be manageable for a period. However, for a person with dementia, their sense of time is broken to them. The concept of deadlines becomes foreign to them. As a caregiver, it is vital and a sign of compassion to look for things to cut out of the schedule and to add in more leisure time. You will find by cutting your loaded schedule down that you can manage their confusion better, and this will reduce the amount of stress and anxiety they are facing.

Slow your day

"It does not matter how slow you go so long as you do not stop." – Confucius

The average day for a person with dementia should almost seem like being on a vacation. The schedule for them should be slow and lose. You must be intentional about making the atmosphere soft and light. The more you can do this for them, the more therapeutic it will be for them, and it will enable them to cooperate more with requests you may have to make of them.

As a caregiver, you will want to create and manage two sets of schedules, one for yourself and the other for your loved one. If you are a fast-paced person, you have to commit to adjusting to your slower speed, when you are present with the one you care for. If you are going to maintain your fast pace, then you will need to incorporate the help of others that have the free time to aid you to maintain a balance.

Practice slowness and patience

"The trees that are slow to grow bear the best fruit." - Moliere

Many people will say they are patient, but when it comes down to it, it is relevant to who they are comparing themselves to. For example, I lived in Michigan and California for an extended period. I can definitively say, that when it comes to traffic, there is a significant difference in attitude for patience in how a person drives depending on what state they are in. I have also spent a significant amount of time in the south, and there is a huge difference in how things get done, and the pace at which it happens. The point is, time and pace is relative.

If you are going to set a gauge for patience, you cannot set the pace as a caregiver; it has to be set by the person you are caring for. You have to manage their care, as well as your life, but remember, they will have lost their since of time, and it will try your patience. So, be observant of what is packed into your day, and make a conscience decision if you should keep something in the schedule or cut it out.

A personal example that I can relay is a situation that developed between my sister and her daughter that she lived with for a season. My niece is very active in her church, and there was a great deal of responsibility that rested upon her. She had a passion for being in church and for connecting with all of her friends. However, her mom had patterns that she remembered when it came to church, which was different than what her daughter practiced. So, when it came time for my niece to leave for church, it became a battle each Sunday trying to get out the door. Those battles caused so much tension and bitterness between mother and daughter. If you desire to have a healthy relationship with your loved one, it is a must that you tone down your schedule.

Know but don't show
"You gotta know when to hold'em, know when to fold 'em, know when to walk away, know when to run." - Kenny Rogers

As a leader, it is important for you to know and manage your schedule and how you will structure the life for you and the loved one that rests in your care. When it comes to agenda, you have to treat it like a game of deception. When I was in the Marines, we used to do a combat drill called the frontal assault. As a fire team, our objective was to come at an objective so hard and fast and with so much force that it would overwhelm the senses and response capability of an enemy to the point that they eventually would fall. This was an upfront, in-your-face way of taking out an enemy combatant.

As effective as that technique is, it is highly ineffective on a person with dementia. If you were to take a direct, frontal approach with them, they would interpret it as a threat. So, you basically have to reduce yourself to pure trickery to persuade them to do things. You will need to plan more time for any task that you need to carry out.

Remember, the brain is slowly dying. The reality of schedules is meaningless and at times, emotionally painful to them. My suggestion to you is to relax, release and relieve to find peace.

Chapter 12 - Communication

"Effective communication is 20% what you know and 80% how you feel about what you know." – Jim Rohn

One of the best tools you can add to your toolbox will be your ability to communicate. Not just with your mouth and how eloquent you can speak. Not just with your ears in how well you can actively listen. I am imploring you to communicate with all of your five senses, along with your empathic spirit. By communicating at this level, you can gain a deeper understanding of what you are dealing with at a given moment and be granted insight on how to take the best response to a given situation.

Tune in

"Abundance is not something we acquire. It is something we tune into." -Wayne Dyer

I do not know if you are of the age where you have experienced or used the old transistor radios. As a kid, I remember there were programs that I would listen to that fueled my imagination while growing up in the 70's. My favorites were *The Lone Ranger* and *Superman.* However, with the old battery operated transistor radios, it was hard to get a clear signal. You would have to wrap the antenna with aluminum foil to enhance the signal. At other times, you would have to maneuver either the radio or yourself to get the signal to come in clear. Those were the days, well before digital or Wi-Fi.

I am relating this to interacting with someone suffering from dementia. They do not have the means to communicate in a steady and clear manner; their brains are all over the map. In some cases, it is never the same day twice even though it seems like they relive events over and over again in their minds. Adjustments are required to communicate or get a clearer signal.

New points of communication

"Communication is a two-way street. Make sure you're willing to listen as much as you're open to speaking." – Unknown

Clear the slate. Everything you know or knew before, allow for it to become irrelevant. Just like your loved one who is trying to fight to maintain a sense of identity and experience a huge change, you too, have to take the new approach. You have to adjust your expectation and remove the assumption that they will understand what you are trying to say. They have too many communication battles they have to address, so to reach them, you have to simplify the communication. You have to communicate through sight, sound, and tactile touch.

In my sister's case, the palms of her hands became very sensitive. What I would do, before I would audibly speak to her, was hold her hand, and with my fingers, tickle the palms of hand. This would make her attentive, so when I spoke, it was a trigger to make her listen. For each person, it will be different. You have to allow yourself to become intuitive. You have to learn to read their body language and bridge a gap to their heart so you can have a stronger means to relate.

Personal interaction

"Be the change that you wish to see in the world." – Mahatma Gandhi

This is where you must remove all assumptions and rules that once existed. Communication, when done in its purest form, is one's ability to express a conscious or subconscious message to another being. There are tons of subtle messages we can give to one another, but when it comes to someone with memory deterioration, you have to be direct, clear, and simple. You have to aim for a heart to heart communication. Your objective should be to help them feel your heart at a slow and personal level.

Word power
"Raise your words, not your voice. It is the rain that grows flowers, not the thunder." -Rumi

As a caregiver, you will need to push yourself to expand and adjust your vocabulary. So, from this point forward, I want you to commit to only using words that have no more than two syllables. The bigger the word and the more syllables, the harder it will be for you to connect with your loved one. Over time, word meanings will deteriorate. You have to simplify your language. Break things down into bite-sized chunks. They will struggle to find meanings of words, so by simplifying your words, you make it easier for them to maintain dignity and self-respect. You defuse stress and, by controlling stress, you lessen the needs for mind-altering, mood-enhancing medication.

Loving touch
"Love is that condition in which the happiness of another person is essential to your own." – Robert A. Heinlein

Early on, I was not an affectionate person. I hated people touching me, hugging me or getting into my personal space. I even struggled with my wife always wanting to hug me. However, for someone helping a person with dementia, you have to become highly conscious of how to use and give loving touches. First of all, remember and respect that everyone has a personal space. Just like a home, you have an appropriate entry point, and you have questionable entry points. For instance, it is usually frowned upon to have your guests enter your home via a side window. That would be highly unacceptable, as with your loved one. You must enter the gate that they manage and stand guard there. You have to approach them, each and every time as a guest would, open and friendly and always through the entry points they establish.

With my sister, you never could touch anywhere on her body unless you touched her hand first. I would have to get her attention verbally, in a soft tone. Then I would reach my hand slowly in front of her, and as she noticed it, she would take it. We would then have a face-to-face conversation before I would proceed to request her to do anything or go anywhere. A lot of the time, to get her to move, I would hug her and then treat our movement as if we were dancing. She would cooperate in rhythm and be happy as if she was having fun. But at all times, I made her feel like she was in control of the contact.

Right ain't right
"If you have to choose between being kind and being right, choose being kind and you will always be right."
– Unknown

I hate being wrong. I will go fight to prove how right I can be. It drives me up the wall to be proven wrong. However, it is a part of life. I have been proven wrong on something that I was so adamant about, on several occasions. It was hard for me to handle. With that being said, imagine how hard it is to receive the reality of how bad things have gotten, how devastating it is to have someone telling you that you are wrong while searching for your foundation and your shifting reality. It can be downright insulting and devastating to who you are and your established identity. It is one thing for someone to point out that you are wrong, but it is an entirely different set of reactions you will have to know that your existence and what you believe may have been fabricated by your imagination.

Our brains are wired to draw conclusions. We have an innate sense of right and wrong, fact and fiction, belief and disbelief. I want to persuade you to tactfully shy away from fighting to be right. There are actual things that exist, and expanded illustrations that may get applied. For a person with dementia, if they are not causing any physical harm to themselves or others, it is all right to let them be right, even when they are wrong. This is especially important when it comes to offenses they may feel have been made against them.

My sister would regularly accuse people of stealing from her. Then I would review the facts and then prove to her that nothing was missing. Many times, things were misplaced and forgotten. But to prove right or wrong simply escalated the situation. I eventually realized that the better approach was not to validate the facts but to validate the feelings. I would apologize to her not for stealing her stuff, but would apologize for making her feel violated. I would do this over and over again until her mind would calm down and let it sink in. I wanted to disassociate her recollection to what happen from her strong emotions about it. If I could keep her stress down, it would gracefully let the moment pass.

Positive affirmation
"Create your day in advance by thinking the way you want it to go, and you will create your life intentionally." - Unknown

For most people, it is hard to take any form of criticism, even if it is constructive criticism. The natural tendency is to become defensive before self-examination. Even the best and strong-willed of us struggle with this. In most cultures, we are programmed to be judgmental and critical of others. We put a little thought in how our opinion and the presentation of that opinion shapes the mood of another. When you are dealing with a person that is experiencing a deteriorating brain, you have to be aware that they do not possess the mental faculty to handle any form of criticism well. They already struggle with their identity, and it is even harder if they feel that people are attacking them for things that are outside of their control.

An excellent way of helping your loved one, while selfishly helping yourself, is to liberally pass out positive affirmation. It works better than most medication to heighten the happiness level and to release the natural chemicals that help them experience joy. Praise them for everything they do right, or even attempt to do right. The better they feel, the better the reaction and interaction you can get out of them.

Being present in the moment

"Accept – Then act. Whatever the present moment contains, accept it as if you had chosen it... This will miraculously transform your whole life." – Eckhart Tolle

In our busy and multi-tasking society, it is very easy to get consumed and busy to a level that we have some difficulties communicating with people's heart. We get preoccupied with agendas and deadlines and in many cases we do a lot, but never stop to examine the cost or even look at *why* we do all that we do. In our multitask society, we have been conditioned to tune out, and tune in at the same time. We can sit at a table with our spouse or sweetheart on a date, and be face-to-face and glued to our cell phones at the same time. We have that urge to seek that so-called momentary distraction. However, it has caused a desensitized generation. We have difficulties relating and having any real and meaningful conversation where we feel like we are being heard or even felt. It is as if our existence could be easily replaced by a Facebook status.

When it comes to people that are in our lives that matter to us, especially if they are suffering from memory impairment, it is very difficult for them to relate to people who are not intuitive to what they are experiencing. You have to be deliberate with being slow in conversation. Listen to what they are saying, but also listen to what they are doing or not doing. Because of the memory impairment, they will struggle to come up with the right words to say, so you have to learn how to ready their body language. Not only do you have to learn how to read them, but you also have to adjust to their frequency so you can find the right way to talk to them. They will listen more with their eyes than with their ears. So that means you have to get face-to-face with them, in a gentle way and speak clearly and softly to them. The sensory pads in their hands will be heightening, and they will learn to experience thing more through tough. If you can hold their hand while talking to them, your message will come across better. Overall, it is important for you to learn how to pick up on their cues so you can equip yourself with the right tools to communicate and listen to your loved one.

Verbal mixed salad
"Laugh at the confusion, smile through the tears and keep reminding yourself that... everything happens for a reason." – Unknown

At an early age, we all are coaxed and encouraged to develop word association. Our left lobe of our brain is where we store words and in the right hemisphere is where we connect words to their definitions. As we learn and grow, we pick up new words, and then practice using them, we store them on the right side of our brain in an understandable order. As a person becomes memory impaired, try to think in terms of "left you lose" and "right you retain." This is the rate of deterioration. A person will lose a word while still having an idea of what that word means. So, when you are dealing with a person with dementia, they will mix up names of people that they know fondly, and they will run through a list of names until they land on a name that feels comfortable to them. My sister once liked an old TV show that was popular in the late 70's called *Good Times*. She had watched it when it originally came out and knew practically every episode.

However, when she wanted me to turn the TV to the station that showed it, she would struggle with it. So she would refer to it as being the "Black People Show." Strange, but funny. It became understandable in her limited capacity to come up with words to express herself.

The power of "thank you"

"We must find the time to stop and thank the people who make a difference in our lives." – John F Kennedy

As I stated earlier, the power of positive affirmation goes a long way. The average person loves praises. If you want to take and keep your loved one on an emotional high, practice praising them with the power of saying "thank you." Be sincere and honest, but also be deliberate and generous in your expression of saying thank you. It will heighten how they feel and condition their attitude into a pleasant atmosphere of response.

In our society, we are being conditioned to say "thank you" less and less. We have a high expectation of everyone and everything and are practicing being disconnected and disrespectful. However, the words of thanks and gratitude were conditioned as a part of basic manners in generations before us, and they still have meaning and power today. Good manners show respect, and when we show another respect, we open the door to receive it multiplied.

"I'm sorry, you're right"

"Apology doesn't mean that you were wrong, or the other person was right. It means that your relationship is more valuable than your ego." -Unknown

Imagine you are in an intense conversation with your loved one. They said some mean and nasty things about you. They accused you of some things that were clearly not true. They may have even told others how bad you had been treating them. The expressions cut you to your core. You begin to question why are you even involved with taking care of them, after all you have done for them. How could they treat you this way? How could this be happening? It is not fair. No matter what you say to them to calm the situation or to right what was wrong, they seem to get madder at you. What can you do to deal with this and the feeling you are having?

As impossible as it may seem, one of the best things you can think about when trying to gain control of a situation is utilizing the power of validation. It is hard to understand that when a person is losing memory, it is on the same level as if they are losing their mind, but they just do not know it. In order to give yourself an advantage over the situation, you have to go overboard with validating their feelings.

There was a time where I argued the fact with my sister. Those were arguments that went nowhere. So I had to implement a strategy where I practiced apologizing to here for how she felt and made her feel okay for feeling the way she did. So, when she accused me of stealing something from her, I would say, "I'm am so sorry that you are feeling upset. I know how I would feel if someone took something that belongs to me. You are right to feel that way. I hope you can forgive me." She would pause and think about it for a moment. Then she would start up again about the same issue. Then I would apologize again for how she felt. Now, for the third time this went on, her feeling died down and she shifted into a more rational state. Now, I am not saying that this will work every time, but it is a good tool to keep handy as you observe things starting to shift in their behavior.

Loving words transform a situation
"I can affect change by transforming the only thing that I ever had control over in the first place, and this is myself." – Deepak Chopra

There is power woven into our vocabulary. We have direct and indirect meanings in the words we choose to use. Our words have the power to build and the power to tear down. Our words have to power to liberate and the power to imprison; the power to bring darkness and the power to bring eternal hope. We can deliver words with volume and words so soft that they almost put you to sleep. We have words that will make us apathetic and some that will get us charged up and off our seats. What I need you to grasp is that there is power in our words, and we have to take ownership of what we say to persuade our environment.

If the person you are caring for is a person that, before their memory impairment, was a person you regularly had harsh words with, you will want to consider strongly developing a new vocabulary for them. Practice a softer tone in your voice. Be deliberate with speaking slower to them. Their brains will struggle with taking in and trying to process too many words. Refrain from harsh, critical expressions. They are going to make mistakes, but you have to be deliberate not to point them out. They will feel embarrassed enough, but to have someone point it out and to rip them apart, is more than their fragile emotion can handle. Practice words of love and encouragement and let that guide the tone for the relationship.

If you have always had harsh words, and that cycle had never been calm, then you may want to consider setting up another caregiver. The problem with the situation is the long term memory. If as far back as they can remember their time with you being harsh, that will only mean they will possess those negative memories when they communicate with you. You have to make a conscious decision to be willing to put up with a lot of verbal backlashes as you care for them, or consider an alternate care provider.

Hold hands and say something honoring

"Be careful what you say. You can say something hurtful in ten seconds, but ten years later, the wounds are still there." – Joel Osteen

It is easy to get caught up with yourself. There is nothing wrong with thinking about one's self. When it comes to making plans for life and thinking about your goals and desires, you have to put good energy into thinking about who you are and where you want to go. It requires a certain kind of love for one's self to put that energy into those thoughts. The risk when we think about ourselves, and that some can dwell on it so much, is that we ignore the fact that there are others in their life. We can allow self-centered thoughts to drive a wedge between people that matter to us.

Over time, many have lost the art of heartfelt communication. It is easier for some to pick up the phone and communicate with others than it is to communicate to the person who is sitting across from us with audible words. Human expression and contact have become demonized in all of the hustle and sufferings that we do to get through life.

There was a time when we knew the value and power of honoring and respecting our loved ones. I remember hearing how it can increase one's health when we practice deliberate and direct honoring of the elders in our lives. It may seem like a chore or a heavy task to do this, but there are liberating and empowering forces involved in openly showing high respect for your loved ones.

A practice that I regularly used to promote peace and to lift my sister's heart when the disease would bring on depression was sitting in a chair, face-to-face with her and this would normally occur after I fed her a meal. I would take her hands and help wash them with a sanitation cloth. I would then hold them and maneuver my head directly into her line of sight. I would then say, "Sis, as much as you drive me crazy, with all that you say and do, I can say, for certain, I still admire you for who you are and how you love and care for your family. Like in the value you bring in all the things you taught us, along the way." She would get a puzzled look on her face because it took a little while for the words to register, but then a beam of peace would spread across her face, and you could see her heart lift. There is power in being willing to go the extra mile to touch the heart of those around you.

Alter some goals

"Setting goals is the first step in turning the invisible into the visible." – *Tony Robbins*

Goals and agenda are important. There is value in life when we can stay organized and meet our given tasks. Life will throw new tasks to us each and every day. We have to plan at times and react to what is going on. If not, chaos will move in and take over, and then we will find life to be out of order and stressful.

When we care for someone who is memory impaired, this becomes a contrasting view. As the impairment increases, you see more and more that they will lose their sense of time and importance of deadlines. They will have brief moments of a strong sense of urgency, but it will be based on erroneous information. However, if you, as a caregiver, keep your schedule at a heightened level, it will cause your loved one to function at a heightened level as well. You will find that the more you can push off your schedule and delegate, the more peace you can bring into your home and promote peace between you and your loved one. It is good and normal to have goals, but you have to separate your drive to meet your goals from that of your loved one.

Offer help instead of just helping

"Never underestimate the difference you can make in the lives of others. Step forward, reach out and help. This week each to someone that might need a lift." – *Pablo*

How would you feel if, as your drove your car to work, someone was waiting for you in the parking lot, so that as soon as you parked your car, they could open it, and help you out of your car? This person would take your bags. They would take you by your hand and escort you to your desk. This same person would linger near, and if you show the slightest sign you were having issues, this person would jump in and help you get your work done. Next, as the day went on, you felt nature calling and you needed to handle business, so you take the walk, and while doing so, this person would accompany you and offer to assist you. Or worse, assist you without asking.

This is an extreme case, but it is an idea of how someone who once had a life and independence feels to have someone come in and with love in their heart, take over their life. We all must understand that no matter how much our loved one may need help, they are still a person that has an identity and that identity has to be respected. Mom never stopped being a mom, simply because she cannot remember that she is a mom. There are things about being the mom that memory cannot control or diminish. There are some things instinctively ingrained in our roles that we play in life. The roles may get a little off in the execution, but nonetheless, the roles are who we are.

We need to be mindful about rushing in to save the day with our approach to help. We need to fight to preserve their dignity as much as possible and for as long as possible. The better we preserve, the better the quality of life will be. We may call ourselves "caregiver," but we have to think like we "care partners." We have to allow our loved ones to lead their life while we gently guide it from behind. We have to refrain from trying to do it all for them and work at being gap fillers for minor areas where they may be falling short.

Listen, connect, agree, and do

"Knowing a person is like music. What attracts us to them is their melody, and as we get to know who they are, we learn the lyrics." – Unknown

How well do your ears work? Not that they just capture sound, but do they listen to what is said and do they listen to what is going on around you? Our ears catch sounds and especially word, but they are symbolic of what we are supposed to capture. We express ourselves; we do so with the intent to plant seeds of memorable moments. Some of us have learned to do this at a heightened level while others of us communicate at a level clouded with static and signal interruption. Either way, we express ourselves because we desire for our existence to matter.

It is a part of our passion as humans also to connect. We do not want to exist merely, but we want to be valuable and vibrant. Many of us express ourselves in a way that when we are present we want people to see and know our hearts and to understand our position. We want to be validated.

One of my sister's greatest frustrations in the later stages of the disease was her passion for mattering and for feeling validated. She felt as if no one understood her and that her thoughts did not matter. She would say on many occasion, "You all think I am crazy and treat me like I don't even matter." Because of the confusion and our passion for helping her staying on track with her memory, our initial handling of things made matters worse in our delivery of care. Instead of trying to correct her, we should have focused on trying to connect with her.

It is not only important to connect but to find a point where you can agree.   Let us say that, in conversation, your loved one is struggling with several points of frustration they are trying to express. Instead of trying to agree and correct on every point, sometimes it is better to agree on the points that you can and excuse the rest. The goal I am trying to move you into is winning by adjusted rules. Understand that you are dealing with a mind with shifting realities. There is no stable ground, so you have to fight for your personal stability while helping them find any form of footing your loved one can stand upon at their current level.

Shift from reactive to responsive
"Pride is concerned with who is right; humility is concerned with what is right." – Ezra T. Benson

I know that growing up, and especially after spending my tour in the military, I developed a heightened reaction to events. I was highly motivated, driven, and dedicated to objectives. I had objectives and agendas. I was observant and attentive to every detail of my life. The motor stayed running, and the eyes were always open. I was conditioned to pounce and to react at a moment's noticed.

I was always the person that was called in the event of a crisis. I was the resident problem solver. I was the go-to guy. Not to say that any of this was bad, but it did present its difficulties when it came to being a caregiver. My personality did not lend to my being sympathetic or empathetic. So I had trouble with reading emotions.

My intense actions were crushing the heart of my sister. My efforts to care for her were exact, to the point, and aggressive. My behavior raised emotions of anxiety and uncertainty that drove her to withdraw and mentally defend herself. She fought for her identity and existence.

Time taught me that I needed to mellow out. I had to step back from who I thought I was, and I also needed to soldier up and adapt to the surroundings and develop a strategy to overcome. So instead of coming at the situation from a tightened, reactive state, I had to shift to being more observant, and ask more questions and get more facts before choosing to move. I learned how to be more responsive to what any given moment was presenting to me. I learned how to slow things down and assess from the heart, before making a snap judgment on what I *think* the situation was, and then let that guide my better action.

Find the message under the message
"Difficulties in life don't come to destroy you, but to help you realize your hidden potential." - Unknown

When communicating with a person with memory impairment, you are not dealing with a black and white situation. Things are psychotic and off the charts at times and at other times, it is a dim shade of gray. This is where your intuitive skills need to sharpen. In life, we are going to get messages expressed to us in all sorts of ways. It may not always come verbally, and it may not come in a clear and neat order. However, if we as caregivers are functioning with a healthy brain, then we have to understand that we have a very powerful tool that works better than most computers on the market. We just have to learn how to tap into its high-level programming.

With an impaired memory, we have to treat every form of communication as if it is a puzzle. We are taking the pieces they are handing us. Figure out where it goes on the puzzle and gently place it where it belongs. But what if they hand you a piece to a different puzzle? What do you do with it? Do you tell them they are wrong and hand the piece back? Here is a thought: instead of trying to help them put together the perfect puzzle, how about playing with the pieces and build an entirely new puzzles. By the time you are done, to the normal eye, it may seem strange and eclectic, but it will build something more beautiful and more valuable than the natural eye can see. You will have built a puzzle that says you love the person you are working with, and the correctness of their memory does not matter, but the bridge to their heart does, and on that bridge, beautiful things happen and it is a place of peace and love, and life happens here.

Get use to cursing and racial slurs and insults
"Always be generous with your encouraging words, you will find they will inspire other to be the best that they can be." – Catherine Pulsifer

This is that "Oh, wow!" moment. It blew me away when I first experienced this from my sister. You see, when growing up, our household was opposites when it came to verbal expressions. My mom was by the book, no nonsense, and respectful with her verbal expression. She said what she meant and was clear and did not use any form of foul language. My father, on the other hand, was a no holds bar, anything goes kind of a person. He said what was on his mind and did not care how he chose to express it. He used practically every curse word in the dictionary, and I think he even invented a few.

My siblings and I got exposed to this on a regular basis. However, we hand a standing rule, where no matter what we heard our father say, we were never to allow to repeat any of it. Foul language was clearly off limits.

Winding the clock forward to when the dementia flared up in my sister, and as the frontal lobe of my sister's brain deteriorated, there went the natural filter that most people have that communicates to us which certain words, phrases, expressions, and jokes are taboo. Being that there was no filter, and, therefore, there was nothing taboo, meant that everything that we experience in our lives, that we learn to lock away and keep prisoner, are now free to roam and become a part of our new expression as if nothing was wrong.

A person with dementia does not look at foul language as being wrong; it is just another word that they still have left in their vocabulary. My sister would cut loose at times, for no good reason. Before the disease, she was respectful with her expression. She may have gotten frustrated at times and may have yelled if she got upset, but as the disease progressed, she would cut loose and could tear into people with the words that she could come up with. After all, it was ingrained in her long-term memory, because she heard countless hours of our father using the same expressions, so, it was foundational to her to use it easily.

Try not to be too alarmed that this will happen. What I found that worked best as a way to redirect that energy was music. The part of the brain that houses our words and expressions take a back seat to what we know as music. When I saw that my sister was getting frustrated and starting to express herself in a less than desirable way, I would either turn on the radio or hum a tune that was familiar to her. She would stop and try to hum along. The music simply misdirected and did an override of the intense situation. So I guess it is true that music does calm the savage beast.

Relationship to your loved one

"Show respect for people who do deserve it, not as a reflection of their character, but a reflection of yours."
– Dave Willis

Even before birth, we are granted a designation. We start out as a child with a mother and father. We also instantaneously become a grandchild, brother or sister, cousin, and in some cases become aunts and uncles. As we grow and traverse life, we pick up other designations. We become friend, buddy, lover, employee, manager, and boss. We develop our identities and personality. Our characteristics expand based on life experiences and our developed responses.

This becomes our identity. Our roles become ingrained in who we are, and we find our identity in our characteristics. This is something we need to think about when it comes to walking through the transition your loved one is facing. They are fighting to hang on to who they are and the many roles that they played. They, as well as yourself, will require a great deal of patience, love, and respect as you work with them daily. It is vital that you help them still fulfill their role to its highest capacity while at the same time gradually adjusting to the transition. If they are your mom, speak to them with the full respect and honor a mom deserves, but function as a partner in that role. Over time, they will respect your support and input, and when the time is right, when they are ready to give up control, the transition will be built on trust instead of force.

Substitution not subtraction

"Too much love never spoils children; children become spoiled when we substitute "presents" for "presence" - Anthony Witham

One of the biggest mistakes I have seen people make when it comes to caregiving is that as soon as they know they have to take care of a loved one, people feel they need to step in, take over, and rearrange their lifestyle. Fair enough, it may be required, but the problem does not rest in what is being done out of love, but in execution. The problem comes in when a loving caregiver makes too many rapid changes in the life of someone who is struggling with parts of their life disappearing. A better tactic to use is to make changes slowly and with the cooperation of your loved one. However, what if things that they have or are engaging in is a detriment to their health and safety? Well, this is where you will implement substitution and subtle deductions. What that means is if they are, let us say, working with sharp objects, but are losing hand-eye coordination, instead of taking it away from them, you swap out the tools or objects they are handling with safer things. You did not tell them to stop, but you are enabling them to live and thrive at a safer level. If after you cooperatively worked with them to adjust to doing something safer, you get push back, your next step would be to subtlety allow for things to disappear. You may even have to use the direct approach, but at the core, you have to keep them safe.

Attract and do not attack

"You attract what you are, not what you want. If you want great, then be great" – Unknown

When noticing something wrong, do not attack the problem. Be intentional about connecting with their spirit and preserving their dignity while correcting the problem. But do not make it appear that they did something wrong. Embarrassment is a powerful emotion. When we are placed in a situation where we are feeling this way, there is a boatload of emotions and thoughts that accompany it. Let us say you spilled your drink all over the table and you are out to dinner with your family in a nice restaurant. Some may say, 'Wow, I'm such a clumsy idiot. How could I have done such a thing? Everyone is looking at me and probably thinking that I am such a dork," or something along those lines. A mature, rational person may be able to assess quickly the situation and find a way to calm their emotion and not draw in false condemnation from others. In most cases, the first reactions of those around you are to stop and try to clean up the mess. However, if a child made the spill, there is something rooted in most kids, that is, they feel like they are *real* failures. Some parents have taken the position that they made a major mistake and scold the child to correct them. Some parents do this from a good place in their heart, but they execute it very poorly. It is not that you tried to correct the matter, but it is in how you corrected. So a child will carry the heavy emotion into adulthood, and then learn how to defensively protect themselves. As maturity sets in, many adults treat mistakes as no big deal, because mistakes are going to happen.

However, when it comes to adults with memory impairments, mistakes are not addressed at the level that a rational adult would handle them; they handle problems like a child would, with deep shame, embarrassment, and defensiveness. When it came to my sister, she had lost her hand-eye coordination. So she became a messy eater. Food would end up all over the place. There were times when I would get after her because her eating area would be a complete mess. However, she would get mad and lash out and defend herself in an aggressive manner. A person with dementia cannot take criticism, so you have to commit to never addressing problems with any form of expressive criticism. Not with words, facial expression, or any sounds of disgust. They can sense that, and it will create barriers between them and yourself, and it will make it harder for you to partner with them for their care and it will destroy any peace you may have.

An alternative is to use subtle distractions to the problem. Such as when my sister would wet on herself and it would leak through her protection. It was messy and smelly, but she had no sense of smell that registered it. She did not even feel that she did this. But, instead of getting mad and blowing up, I had to address the situation creatively. I simply said to my sister that it has been a "Hot day and that it was a long day." Then I also told her that I had a new outfit I wanted her to try on, but I needed her to shower before I would let her play dress up. Once she thought about it, she quickly perked up and willfully went to the shower, with assistance from my lovely wife, and got cleaned, while I took care of the furniture that got wet. The problem got addressed without us having to escalate the emotions, and this preserved her dignity. Yes, it was work on my wife and myself, but this was less work than having to deal with defeated emotions and uncontrollable outburst. We had to pick the lesser of two evils to produce a better outcome.

Do not make it make sense

"The only way to make sense out of change is to plunge into it, move with it, and join the dance." – Alan Watts

"Just go with it." Know this phrase and add it to your thoughts and vocabulary. This is the part of caring where you get to have a little fun. You see, when it comes to our memories and memory storage process, the events that happen in a given day are not all that we see. Even in a healthy brain, we have the ability to subconsciously embellish and twist the perspective of facts. You could get three people and have them look at the same object and have each describe something different. This is because the brain will fill in the gaps of our personal logic center and develop our understandable interpretation of what we think to happen.

A person with memory impairment is a bit worse. They have a declining short-term memory. Recent events they have experienced become limited where memories are stored due to the breakdown in synaptic nerves and memory brain cells. There is no place for the detail of that memory to absorb. That which they can remember gets mixed in with other memories they have, and then they developed a spliced view of reality.

In my sister's case, she was big in knowing our family tree, history, customs, and traditions. She collected all sorts of memorabilia and wrote down dates and events that involved our family members. She would meet with family members and talk about family history when she was healthy. However, later in her disease, with a portion of her memory gone and eyesight failing, it was increasingly hard for her to distinguish facts from fiction. Unfortunately, on my father's side of the family, many of the males look alike. She would look at me and confuse me with our father or our grandfather or one of our great uncles or cousins. After a while, I would play along and pretend to be the person she thought I was. Then after a while of carrying on a conversation, I would say, "Where is that $5 you owe me?" She would stop and think back to if she did owe $5 and then her mind would shift back to reality and get a laugh out of it.

What I discovered is that there is no harm in her being factually wrong, just as long as she is not causing harm to herself or to anyone else around her. The risk came in when she had to talk to people who did not know she had dementia, such as if she had to go to the hospital. I had to warn others about it, and if they were trained to handle it, then I would let them interact. If they did not meet my standards of experience, I would have to interpret the fact for her. But for the most part, I had to just give way to where her brain was at the moment so we could have peace in our relationship.

Where have all the people gone?

"Do you want to be happy? Let go of what's gone, be grateful for what remains and look forward to what is coming." – Unknown

When I started to take care of my sister many years ago, I had so many people step up and commit to being there and to help out with whatever was needed to address the needs of my sister. The early years were manageable, but as the disease progressed, bit-by-bit, people began to step away, and the help became scarce. It upset me to have people, who was seeing her struggle and to see me struggle with how I had to care for her, systematically drift away.

Many who stopped helping just gradually made their absence happen over time by cutting down their frequency of visits. Others sited life events as their reason for declining to help. To me, it was hurtful because I was in the trenches and needed the help. I was angry and becoming judgmental over the situation, and this was causing riffs in the family.

After an interaction with wellness coach on this matter, I was given a better strategy on how to address this situation. Instead of passing judgment and expressing anger, I was granted permission to ask questions. The questions enabled me to gain clarity as to why they were not helping and by discussing it, I gave the other family members a chance to be clear, open, and honest, and I was allowed to focus on liberating them. In this way, they were free to help out of love, versus helping out of guilt and condemnation.

My sister had three children. As the disease ramped up, one of her sons had trouble with coming to see her. As her prognosis got worse, the situation forced me to have a conversation with that son. I was initially upset with him for living so near to her, but choosing to make his presence so scarce. My interaction with my sister was an act of kindness and mercy. It took a lot of time and patience. It was no easy task. Now, I am not tooting my own horn, but I am expressing that what I did was not just support, but a spirit of connection, something that her son should have been experiencing with her. So, I had to ask, for his sake, "Why are you feeling trouble about not spending time with your mother?" I did not want to put him on the defensive or accuse him of anything, but I wanted to give him room to express his feelings. I was giving him room to express any underlining reasons for his choosing to step back.

I also had to take the high road, for health sake, in allowing him to step back from being involved. My pushing him to get involved was creating stress all around. It was causing me to work hard to pull him in, as well as rely on him. It was disappointing to experience the let down when he did not follow through. I released him from care so it would not cause emotional stress for my sister. She could sense when people were around who did not care and she allowed her emotions to express her dissatisfaction with it.

Bottom line, you have to be fully willing to release someone from service who is not passionate about being there. It does no real service or satisfaction to the level of care to have someone there that is not caring or is distracted or holding animosity or emotionally struggling with seeing their loved one in that way. The best thing to do is to release the stress. Bless and release them and move on.

Do not throw out food or things when the loved one is present

"Respect people's feelings, even if it doesn't mean anything to you. It could mean everything to them." – Unknown

When you are in a living situation with a person struggling with mental impairment where they once lived alone prior to the disease, please understand that they will struggle with a sense of smell and taste. This is especially true when it comes to food and food quality. They may not really know when food has gone bad from sitting in the fridge too long. Out of the kindness of your heart, you will notice the issue by opening the fridge and being hit by the foul odor. The first urge is to pull the garbage can over and go to work clearing the fridge. However, the risk is very high that they may take it as an offense. For some, this is a level of security for which they will want to manage in agreement with their lifestyle. So, out of respect, your first approach should be to let them notice that you see that the date has expired on certain things, or show them the mold on the food, then offer to assist by helping them clean their fridge. However, some may have the hoarder mentality. If that is the case, stop right there! What you will have to do is coordinate getting access to their house while they are out. You will then need to clean the fridge in their absence. You may want to take it a step further by getting replacement fresh food. Also, for any food that will remain in the fridge, try to maintain the positioning order, so they will have an idea of where to find things when they have to go back in there. It will reduce the confusion and any anxiety they may experience because you came and changed their refrigerator and at the same time destroyed their little world.

Fight, flight or fright

"What you hold in your mind on a consistent basis is exactly what you will experience in your life." – Tony Robbins

Fight, flight or fright. These are an automatic and autonomic reaction. In this section, we will cover how your actions can trigger any of these responses when a problem shows up. The average person, when faced with a scary situation, will either choose to fight (stand up for themselves) or flight (RUN!) or be in fright (find some place to hide until the storm blows over). With a healthy brain, we can usually examine a situation and give an appropriate response. In some cases, it can be very predictable what the response will be. If there was w fire, the natural response would be to either put it out or get out. Pretty simple, right? However, with a person with a memory impairment, the reactions may not always be what you think. While the brain is deteriorating, it is at the same time fighting to make sense of what their eyes, ears, smell, taste buds and fingertips are experiencing. The logic they once had no longer makes rational since. Their brain is filling in the blanks, and in some cases, making fact out of fiction.

So, what does this mean? When it comes to how you are relating to your loved one, you need to think about the end outcome you want, and slowly entice them to get there. I have found that the direct approach appears threatening to many. When you give someone with dementia a direct command, they take it as you bossing them around very easily. This will lead to a conflict that could easily blow out of proportion. Tread lightly. You have to become "Disney" to them. You have to make them feel like you are the happiest place on earth. You have to become lights, and glitter, and the reason they want to get up in the morning. Just like people have this burning desire to go to *Disneyworld*, you have to create that kind of atmosphere emotionally for them so they can respond to your direction without them knowing you are leading them.

Invite partnership - finding your place to serve
"Life's most urgent question is: What are you doing for others?" – Martin Luther King Jr

I have said this on a few different occasions, but for many, they look at what they are doing for their loved one as a form of caregiving. However, that term conjures up a lot of negative mental connotations. We can tend to feel like servants in a thankless job. Long term, this can become mentally and emotionally draining and can become almost hopeless, if you are not mindful.

It takes a great deal of compassion to do this kind of work. It takes a strong, elevated attitude of love to have what it takes to carry it through to the end. But I want to give you another spin on how to look at this. Many of us would not willfully become a slave to anyone for any reason. But if you told me that I had to give up a third of my blood with the knowledge that I was giving something that could be a cure to save thousands of lives I would give more. I would feel like I was partnering with whoever came up with the concept of that cure.

When it comes to caring for our loved one, we need to think in terms of being a partner with them. We may have the noble goal of fighting for a cure, or engaging in the prolonging of their life and giving them the highest level of health, or we may be partnering in their care in a way that preserves their dignity when they no longer can defend themselves from themselves. Either way, as a partner, you have to make yourself aware of where they are at and gain their permission to assist. When they let you in to work with them, you get so much more out of the relationship than you do by pushing your way into their lives and their space.

Capture moments
"Everyone here has the sense that right now is one of those moments when we are influencing the future." –
Steve Jobs
This is probably going to be one of the most fun and rewarding projects you could ever do for your loved one that will benefit you as well as them with preserving and enhancing some of their memory. By the time I was able to engage with my sister on this matter, her memory and motor skills were too far gone for me to effectively do this in video form, so I ended up doing this in print. I will explain that a little later. This is something you will want to get a jump on, and you do not have to be scared to do. You do not have to be tech savvy to do this, nor do you need any special equipment to pull this off.

You will need a video recording device. Do you have a cell phone or a smartphone? That is all you need for this first part. Figure out how to make a simple video recording. That is all the main technical know-how you need. What shall you record? First of all, think of what is interesting to them. Is it their kids; their job? What projects have they volunteered to perform? People they love? Hobbies? Friends? Pets? Whatever it may be, think of interesting questions you can ask that can get them to talk about their interests.   A conversation started could be: "Can you tell me about the time, when you first met your husband?" This will cause their mind to reflect, and it is a wonderful thing to watch their face as their mind spins back to that pleasant moment, and they bring it forward.   As they answer, record the event.   It may not be accurate, but that is okay.   It is the frame of reference that they have at that moment and the best point of stability that they possess at the time.   The important thing here is to get them comfortable talking.   Ask as much as they can handle at a given moment.   Do not overwhelm them with too many questions or types of questions that make them feel uncomfortable.   You want them to feel at ease so that they can express more.

Once you have a few recordings made, you can then move to the next step—putting them in DVD format or a format that is reasonable enough for you to play back to them.   Some of you may have tablets that you can use to play video for your loved one, but I am recommending DVD because this is something that you can load and then place in a continuous loop that can play over and over again without intervention.

On a Mac, you can use software called iMovie or on a PC you can use Moviemaker.   Both are free, built-in software.   You can transfer the video files you made into a folder on that system and format the movies and edit the view and sound quality.   Once you have done a nice editing job, you can then burn them to a blank

DVD. After which you can take the DVD and play it for your loved one from time to time. This will help reinforce their memories, and it will give you a memento and a strong reference point of who they once were.

With my sister, when here health was failing, and she could no longer talk, I was then forced to do some research on her life, and I wrote a biography on her. I detailed everything I could think of, and I gathered information from other family members and friends so that I could have a good composite of who she was. I then printed it up on some very nice, high-quality paper. My sister was in a nursing home at the time, and she was bedridden. She could not speak, move, or do anything for herself and she was at the mercy of the staff most of the time. I interacted with the staff daily. So to enhance my interaction, I took this writing I made and posted it on the wall over her bed, in clear sight. I wrote it in such a way that when visitors and workers read it, they got to look inside the person they were treating. I wanted them to view her as more than just a patient, but as a person who lived, loved, and mattered. The staff loved the expression, and it resonated with their hearts and in a way, it helped improve the relationship with the other patients that the staff had to care for. Overall, it was a powerful connecting point for me. It enhanced my thinking beyond a superficial level. It also pushed me to think deeper on my life and the legacy that I will leave. It taught me to cherish the moments and the people while I have them. It also taught me not just to have memories, but to make memories and to never underestimate the impact that I may have on the lives of others.

Do not tell them what not *to do*

"Respect people's feelings, even if it doesn't mean anything to you. It could mean everything to them." – Unknown

Have you ever encountered a person who is strong willed? Consider a child who is strong in thought and determined on what they want to do. When comes to getting that child to stop, you almost have to move deep into the physical level to persuade them not to do something that they are adamant about doing. It is pretty bad with a child but is really bad when you are dealing with a full grown adult.

I have found that to tell someone with dementia what they cannot do can lead to a lot of resistance, especially if it is something they have done out of habit for a long time. Their skills may not be as sharp anymore, so the task has become difficult. What if that task is something that is risky and could potentially harm himself or herself or someone else? How do you get them to stop? Telling them, "no" will simply cause them to dig in. And to use clear logic with them may not work, based on where they are at with their mental and emotional states. So what do you do?

1. Connect - First of all, on a continuous basis, whenever you interact with your loved one, you must communicate verbally, emotionally, respectfully, and with body language, at a heart level. It cannot be you giving orders all the time, but it has to be you showing that you care and that their feelings matter. If you are not passionately willing to connect, you will not

have the means to give them room to respect you or anything you say or may request of them.

2. Partner – You are going to hear a lot about this. It is what we are doing. We are coming alongside them and letting them know that they are not alone and that they have people that care about them or what they are trying to do in life and assisting them with getting the best out of the rest of their life. Through partnering, you build trust and respect.

3. Redirect – When witnessing your loved one struggle with performing a daily task, you are inclined to assist. However, stay observant. Think independence. Is there a way you can scale it back or break it up into smaller, manageable chunks? If they are adamant about it, such as driving, then how could you redirect them? Ask thoughtful questions, such as "I'm confused. Can you tell me why do you need to drive to the store? Is there something I can assist you with getting? I am happy to go with you, or I would love to drive you and spend time with you. Would that be okay?" Ask questions that give them alternatives that look more appealing than what they originally had in mind. What I am getting at is that the thought they have of driving is on a patterned track, and what you have to do is interrupt that track and come up with something that is an alternative with more rewards. Not only offer to drive them to their destination, but also offer to drive them to a special secret location that you turn into a

surprise. Let them know that it can only happen if they let you drive.

4. Separate – Let us say your loved one is adamant about driving. This is something they will not give up. Well, in my sister's case, she was a dangerous driver in her advanced stages of her disease. So what I had to do is one day while she slept, I had her car moved to a location that was out of sight. When she woke up the next morning, she went to look for her car and then she was upset that it was not in its spot. I had told her that it was leaking fluid, and I had to put it in the shop. She was upset that it was gone but happy that it was being taken care of. This went on for several days. Then after about a week, I told her that the car was so bad and beyond repair that they had to total the car. She was not happy, but it gave her terms she could understand and live with. So, from that point forward, she gave up the idea of driving. And she was fine with it at that point. I did not have to tell her no or what she could not do. I simply placed it in better terms where she could understand, given her limited frame of reference. I put it in terms that we both could relate to.

The power of a clear and consistent apology
"Never ruin an apology with an excuse." – Kimberly Johnson

I want you to imagine the work that a farmer has to do. They have to work the ground daily. They have to till it, weed it, sow seed, water it, and harvest it. When it comes to the human mind of one person to another, it is in a similar fashion that we have to approach things. When it comes to farming, the rule is that what you put in is what you get out. So if you want peace, calm, and pleasantry to come from the person you are interacting with, then you have to sow a lot of that seed into that person. Bear in mind that you may be sowing seed into a mind that has not been tilled or weeded. It may be difficult for that mind to produce a good yield.

When dealing with a mentally impaired mind, you have to understand that this is a mind that was once cultivated and fertile. But over time, sections of the land have been poisoned and rendered unable to produce any good yield. However, there are sections that are still functioning. In those sections, you need to fertilize and plant seed and nurture and protect that field for as long as it can produce. Specifically, in the area of perceived offense, a person with dementia can easily be ticked off because they are losing their grip on reality. They will blame the nearest person around for anything that seems to be out of place. As I stated before, you may have to play along with their delusions and take the hit and not fight to be right. However, one of the best seeds you can sow to help combat this is that of an apology. If you can practice using this when tensions are running high and use it as a tool to control the barometer of emotions, you will find it to be quite effective.

When I say apologies, I do not mean to admit you did wrong. What you are apologizing for is how they are feeling when they are in their unpleasant mood. You may not be able to change their situation or their thought about you, but you do have the power to let them know you care about their feelings and that you will do what it takes to make it right. For the most part, this works very effectively to calm a lot of tense situations. You may need to do this a few times in a single setting to get emotions at a reasonable level.

Always adjust the tone of voice
"People may hear your words, but they feel your attitude." – John C. Maxwell

What you put out is what you are going to get back. Even if you are a person in authority over another, we all must understand that there is a law of attraction. Therefore, if we are a violent person, we will draw violence into our lives. If we are a deceitful person, we will draw deceit into our dealings with others. If we are passionate about life, we will draw people into our lives that are just as passionate.

When it comes to the vocal tones that we use, we have to be mindful that a person with dementia has audible issues developing. They develop an overactive imagination, and they will hear voices from the past that are constantly playing in their head at varying volumes. When you speak, your voice has to compete against that. The tendency is to raise your voice when you feel no one is listening. However, that just aggravates the situation. What I found very effective is to soften your tone and to practice smiling when speaking. Exercising the muscles that make you smile impacts the tones you use when talking to others. It also helps to release stress and endorphins in your brain. Another effective strategy I learned was to put a rhythmic tone in my voice to the point of almost singing. What I discovered is that there are portions of the brain that deeply connect with music. When a person hears music they can more easily relate to the soothing rhythmic tone. It will move them to a calmer state of mind, and you will have a better reception with what you are saying.

Saying "calm down" does not work
"Don't make me mad then tell me to calm down. That's like shooting someone and then wondering why they are bleeding." – Unknown

When I am emotionally hot, telling me to calm down has the opposite effect. I do not calm down on command. I calm down because I know and feel that it is the right thing to do. That comes after the issue has been addressed either through correction of the action or me venting my emotion. Most of the time I have my emotions keyed in on why I am upset and what satisfaction means. There are also times when my train goes off the rails, and I am coming in hot and fast. It is hard to hold back a person coming in at full blast.

So, what do you say? What do you do, especially with a person with memory impairment? First of all, you have to assess the situation and surroundings. Are you in a public or private settings? Are you at a social function or a family gathering? If you are in a private setting, it will be easier to address the situation. If there is a flair up in public, then you will want to move to a private setting as fast as possible. If their emotions are playing out in front of an audience, it could quickly escalate to a point that you may not be able to direct. If they got wound up around the family who are keyed into the situation and health condition, then you may be a little safer, and they may be of value to assist you in calming the situation.

But by no means, should you say the words, "calm down." They will interpret it as you dismissing their feelings and emotions. They will think you are not validating their existence. When you get them into a calmer setting, what you need to do first is calm yourself and, if possible, take a seat. Say something like, "It's been a long day. My feet are tired. Do you mind if I sit down while you tell me what has you upset?" This will invite them to move to an emotionally calmer setting. Next, I would acknowledge how they feel by saying, "I can see that you are upset. I am very sorry you feel uptight. I don't like that I (or whatever it may be) has caused you to feel this way. Can you tell me what I said that made you get so upset?" At that point, you set the framework for them to express themselves and you are telling them that you care about how they feel.

People want to be respected and to matter. When our minds are playing tricks on us, it is easy to feel like everyone is out to get us. It is not right or fair, and we want satisfaction. But we must understand that calmness can only come after the storm has run its course. What we have to do as a caregiver is adjust our sails as we navigate the sea of chaos, so that we can survive the storm and try to keep everything intact during the process. Allow them room to express themselves, but put it in a context where they cannot harm themselves or anyone else. Once they get a chance to vent, the storm will pass.

Three is a crowd
"Pick your battles. You don't have to show up to every argument you're invited to." – Mandy Hale

Pulling in another person into a disagreement with a person with memory impairment is a huge no-no. My experience has taught me that this simply escalates the situation. Your heart may be in the right place because you wanted support and confirmation of what you are experiencing. You want to state the facts, and you want this addressed in a rational and logical manner. However, you are playing against a stacked deck. Do not fight to be right, but fight to be reasonable. Right is wrong in mental impairment. You have to see that bringing in a third party only communicates that you are ganging up on the person with the memory issue. They will automatically feel threatened and will fight and push back harder. It is better to think ahead of time of strategies on how to navigate away from or to channel the agitated energy. I will say it again, refrain from pulling in a third party unless things have gotten physical and you need help to keep your loved one from hurting you, others, or themselves.

Intentionally practice and talk about their good old days

"Let us never know what old age is. Let us know the happiness time brings, not count the years." – Ausonius

Our minds are a powerful storehouse of information and events. The events we experience are reference points to key moments of life. For many of us, we can remember moments where we did something that gave us confidence and hope. Moments that made us cry, but filled out hearts with great joy. Some of us will remember our first date and the place where we met, and the clothes we wore and taste of the food we ate. Our minds recorded the moments like when our child was born and the first time we held them in our arms. I remember the first time I flew in a plane. It was thrilling and scary for me, all in one. I remember playing baseball with my parents when I was a small child. My dad pitched the ball to me, and I hit it over the backyard fence. \

Moments like these have left an indelible impression on our hearts, and it goes into the making of who we are. As you care for your loved one who is struggling with the memories they are losing, it is extremely important to engage them in conversation and activity that allows them to reflect on memories that they still possess. Take time to jot down what they are saying about things they used to do, people they knew, and places they went. You will want to get pictures of those events if they are available. This helps reinforce what memories they still do have, and it supports pieces they are missing. This plays a major role at keeping them calm and reducing their anxiety. Please bear in mind, the more anxious they become, the faster the symptoms will progress. The faster the symptoms, the harder it will be for you to manage their care. Even if you are doing at-home care or utilizing the services of assisted living or nursing home.

I would also suggest you invest in video and audio recordings of things that reminds them of their youth. It helps with giving them a reference point of clarity. It blesses and gives peace and reassurance to your loved one in that you care for them, and you are helping them maintain their memories. It also enables you to get to take a deeper look into the person you are caring for and will enable you to learn some things that just might impress you about who they are.

❖Chapter 12 - Communication❖

Do not correct errors

"The only way to make sense out of change is to plunge into it, move with it and join the dance." – *Allen W. Watts*

Hanging loose. Take it easy. Do not sweat the small stuff and trust me. It is all small stuff. I remember reading in Dale Carnage's *How to Win Friends, and Influence People,* that you should not correct other people for the sake of the relationship. That means volumes when it comes to a person struggling with memory issues.

You will find that they are wrong on facts more times than they will be right. The natural urge is to say, "I don't think you are correct" or "I think you have some of your facts mixed up." Those types of statements made to a person struggling with memory issues can be emotionally devastating. The average person has means to rationalize and analyze what you said in a way of correction. However, what happens when there is no logic or reasoning? A person struggling with memory issues will take it as a personal assault and will fight tooth and nail to defend their position.

What I had to adopt as a rule to address this was first to assess and see if the statement or action would harm anyone. If there were no harm, then I would choose never to correct an off-fact. My goal had become to protect my sister's dignity and to enhance our relationship. My point was not winning an argument, but to not have a reason to have an argument. Peace has to be the primary order of the day. If I allow stress and frustration to be a regular part of the day, then I can also expect to shorten their life expectancy and devalue the quality of their life.

Do something with them instead of just talking to them
"They will forget what you said but will not forget how you made them feel." – Carl Buechner

Your time is valuable. There are deadlines and demands that call on you and take away your time. There are schedules that are thrown at you all day long and, for the most part, you find yourself moving to the beat of a drum that your schedule or other people's schedules make for you.

Your loved one with the memory issues is a person of their former self. They had skills and hobbies that defined who they once were. For some, it is painful to watch the transition. They cannot do what they used to do. They struggle with day-to-day tasks. Frustration comes easily to them. So, what do you do to help? Time! Give them your time. I am not saying give them a ton of your time, but what I am saying is give them some of your focused, undivided time. Get face-to-face, hand-to-hand, knee deep involved and blessed them with your presence. If they like crafts, then take about 30 minutes and work with them and do some crafts. If they like flowers, then take 30 minutes to an hour to work the ground and plant some flowers. If they liked to work on motors, then take some time to assist them with this task. Do not shoot for perfection. Shoot for connection and time. They do not necessarily need to do the stuff; they need to connect with you. So, break them off a piece of your valuable time.

Remember that their brain is dying as well as lying to them

"Appearances are often deceiving." – Aesop

That heading may seem cruel and disheartening, but we all must come to terms with what is happening. However, in life, it is not what is happening to us that matters as much as how we choose to respond to it. In all honesty, from the moment of birth we have been placed on a path that will eventually lead to death. There is no age limit on it, or income, race, or religious belief that protects us from this fact. Death is a part of life that will always remain with us.

I want to do my best to try to help you relate to a person who is experiencing brain death. Not only from what they are experiencing but from what you experience as you watch them go through this. This will be one of the hardest things you may ever have to go through.   As the early stages of the memory loss progress, you will see gradual changes. The changes will impact the content and validity of what they are saying to you. Their speech pattern may change. Some will begin to repeat themselves or even stutter. Later in the disease, you will see some may even lose the ability to speak because of the deteriorated portion of the brain that has the words or that control the motor skills to move the mouth.

I also noticed that the facts will not always line up to reality. As a caregiver, this part can be one of the most frustrating. You may be seeing a person that looks healthy, and engaging in life, but when you talk to them at an in-depth level, you begin to experience that what they are expressing may be off or even out of place. In some cases, it may come off as being out of character or offensive. You must understand that with the memory loss, to them it feels like they are under emotional attack, and they are using their twisted representation of the facts to fight back for a part of themselves that was taken away. So please try to give them room and give yourself a mental break from trying to be right and focus more on trying to find ground on where you can connect.

Use nursery rhyme books
"Music and rhythm find their way into secret places of our soul." – Plato

I just recently became a grandfather for the first time. I am so excited about it. I never thought that I would feel this way about anyone, but I can honestly say, as tiny as my granddaughter's hands are, she has me wrapped around those tiny little fingers, and I have her wrapped around mine. I love to sit and sing and read to her. She gets so excited when I do this. Her eyes light up, and I can see those little wheels turning as I try to communicate. Her brain is connecting to me at the simplest level. I open the book, show her pictures, and I illustrate the sounds of what the picture is saying with voices that match the settings. I allow myself to have fun, which then enables her to have fun.

With that same level of energy, creativity, and fun, I was able to find a way to connect with my sister. I had to simplify things down to nursery level. I would say the beginning of nursery rhymes that I think she would know and then pause, and wait for her to fill in the blanks. So, I would say something like, "The wheels on the bus go ....." or "Humpty Dumpty sat on a wall, Humpty-Dumpty had a great fall. All the king's horses and all the king's men, ..." I used these to connect with the base memories she still obtained and enabled her to use them, and that would in turn help her engage other parts of her brain and improve the overall health of how she functioned day-to-day.

Watch and diffuse the snappy comeback
"Kind words can be short and easy to speak, but their echoes are truly endless." -Mother Teresa

As a kid, I would watch a lot of sitcoms. One of my favorites was an old TV show called *Good Times.* Some of my favorite moments were when the lead character, JJ, would get into a heated discussion with his sister, Thelma. They would rip into each other all the time and for the most part, for no good reason other than sibling rivalry. It was fun and games and the laugh track made it seem lighthearted. People outside of TV try to carry on life in the same way. It does not matter if it is between siblings, spouses, friends, or co-workers, we can be rude in our expressions for the sake of a joke, to the point where we cannot see how deep we are cutting into someone's spirit. It requires an intuitive spirit to be able to see when your cutting remarks start to leave scars. People do not always say when they are hurting. Some hurts run deep before they can surface. For healthy people, it may take a while before you hit that last nerve. With someone with memory impairment, it may only take a little push to move him or her over the edge.

I have heard people say to others, "What's wrong? You can't take a joke?" This is a common expression we give after we have said or done something that was intentionally designed to be hurtful, but we mask or wrap it in humor as an escape clause. I want to help elevate the level of thinking. Practice pulling back on the jokes and try to be real and honest with people. In actuality, try to practice slowness. We tend to be short and dismissive with other people when we should work at cherishing life's vital moments. When it comes to caring for your loved one, hold off on being short and giving snappy comebacks to them. Each time you do it, it diminishes their spirit and self-worth.

Do not say "it's okay" because it is not
"Honesty does not always bring a response of love, but it is essential to it." – Ray Blanton

I am losing my mind and freaking out, and someone comes and says, "it's okay." How is it okay, that I know I placed my keys in the same spot that I always have, and I searched high and low for them and cannot find them? I ripped my house apart to find them, and I practically accused everyone of stealing them and then I made myself late for work because I could not find my keys. I then open the regenerator door to get some cold water and there, sitting by the orange juice, are my keys.

What I described is very common for most people. Our brains are firing off thousands of thoughts at once. Our body and mouth cannot even keep up with all the things we think of in a given moment. At times, we get thoughts jumbled and confused. Some of those complex thoughts lead to confusion and frustration. We act on things that we thought we were sure of, and then it turns out that we could not have been more wrong. I am expressing this from the point of view of a person with a healthy brain.

Now think of it from the perspective of a person who is suffering from mental impairment. Would it not be a little bit more overwhelming? Even threatening, because it seems like it is happening more often and with more and more critical things. If you are in that position, you may even engage in an act that may have caused harm to you or another. Or if you are that person, you may be under the care of another. Now think, how is it okay that you just ran your car into a tree in the middle of your yard? For many of them, fear and frustration dominate their thinking. They are in a situation where they are having an out of body experience. It is as if they are waking up in a strange place with strange people every day and they are trying to react to their surroundings and make heads or tails of what is in front of them.

What works best is to connect patiently with their emotions and, through facial expression and body language, let them know that they are safe and have plenty of room to make mistakes. Let them know that they are loved and appreciated, no matter what. What they are going through is not okay, but you can put out the emotional projections that it is all right, and this will create room for them, and you, to feel better in spite of the circumstances.

How do we connect and communicate?
"When someone else's happiness is your happiness, that's love." -Lana Del Rey

From one animal to the next, communication is a gift granted to each of us, by the Creator. We have a multitude of messages to transmit to each other in a variety of ways. It seems even today that we are inventing more and more ways to connect and relate to one another. It is not a bad thing in itself. However, with our advanced communication we have limited ourselves in how we connect.

Connection is something that happens at a deep emotional level. This is the point where you are relating heart-to-heart. It is where you deeply understand what another is saying, and you are feeling it at the same time. This level of communicating places you in an empathic state. It comes not from the words you say or if they were heard, but it is in how it is delivered. Paying special attention to the tone and pitch of the voice. Eye contact and response also enhances communication, as well as active listening, where you are either asking deeper questions about a statement or stating back what you understand.

When a person feels heard and like their life matters, they respond better and it reduces stress. It was my aim to keep my sister's stress level as low as possible. She struggled in this area, but I also witnessed that the higher her stress went, the faster her memory loss symptoms emerged. So I had to work at slowing things down and relating to her at her lowest level. It did not stop or slow down the disease, but it did help me to understand her heart, and it placed a level of joy and trust in her that she could feel comfortable to express and relate. Overall she felt love and respect.

Public (see), personal (talk), and intimate (touch) space
"When you touch someone's heart, they will never quite be the same again. Part of your life will live with them always." – Unknown

One of the things that happened to my sister that hurt her and made her feel disrespect was when she was in her nursing home, and it was the designated day that they showered the patient. She was already upset that she had to go through an adjustment for her living arrangement, and she hated that she lost her freedom and power of choice. It made it worse when she was told that she had to take a shower with the help of a stranger. She took it as a threat. When this event occurred, she fought. She fought back hard. She was scared and felt threatened, so she punched the nurse and orderly who were trying to forcibly undress her. This led to her being admitted to a psych ward so they could put her on stronger meds to control her mood swings.

In reality, what she was experiencing was not mood swings, but it was cause and effect. I can from experience say that the training has to be enhanced and refined by workers as they address the needs of a dementia patient. Dementia patient care is not "one size fits all." There are, still some basics things that need to be addressed when it comes to personal space. When it comes to all human beings, we have what we call our public space. That is what we see with our visual eyes and what we allow others to see. We have an unwritten rule on what we call our boundaries. No one can just come in and invade it. The next layer of access to our personal space is our verbal and audio engagement. Out another way, this is how we initiate conversation and the way we listen and respond to what is being said. This also occurs at the written level. I see a lot of personal interaction when it comes to social media, such as Facebook or Twitter. We then move deeper into an intimate level when we touch. Our touches say a lot about what we are trying to communicate. Each touch has a separate message. There is a difference in what is being said when we touch someone's hand versus rubbing their shoulder. There is a deeper level of communication taking place when the torso area is touched, and especially in the genital area. When we break things down to their basic animal instinct, when our genitals are touched, it is related to a sexual act. For a person dealing with mental impairment, some may interpret that in an aroused or defensive manner, based on the circumstances. So it is extremely important, that if you are going to be the position to touch your loved one's persons, then you must do it in stages.

First, make audible contact. Let them know you are there. Be a friendly face that they can relate to. Be a soft, inviting voice that their spirit can connect to. All of this must be done before the first touch. Second, the first place you always touch is the hand. Extend your hand slowly but in an exact manner, as if to shake their hand. This is basic human contact 101. If we see a hand extend, we take it to shake it. The next stage is your conversation. Based on the level of memory loss, it is not always advisable to take the direct approach with what you are trying to get them to do. You have to leave bread crumbs that lead up to the end results. So, first of all, if they have not washed for a while, maybe you can talk about the weather and how hot it feels. They may not feel physically hot, but you can get them to feel hot, by talking about how hot it is and how sweaty it makes you feel. Or you can talk about how nice they look, but also about an event that is coming up, and how nice it will feel to get dressed up for it. Through those two suggestions, you can get the wheels turning in the right direction. Gradually persuade them to change clothes. You will want to start talking about how refreshing it will be to get a nice shower. But before doing that, you can talk about a new soap that you have and rave about how good it smells. Then you will want to ask them how they would feel if they tried it out. You will want to put things in the form of simple questions that they will be willing to answer.

Next, you will want to adjust the phrases and verbal suggestions so that it will make them feel as if it was their idea to get washed. Get in the habit of asking, "What do you think about...?" So, for instance, ask, "What do you think about this soap, do you think it will help you smell fresh?" Or "What do you think about the temperature of the water, will that be too warm for you or do you need it to be a little colder?"

Bear in mind that all of these questions are taking place well before you start assisting them with getting undressed. Now when you are ready for them to start undressing, you will want to say, "Can I assist you with unbuttoning or unzipping your clothes to help you get ready for your shower?" You want them to grant permission first. Second, you want to take their hand and guide it over the buttons or zipper and assist them with the motions. They will more than likely lose dexterity, so it will turn into you doing it for them. However, you want their hand there, so it seems and feels like they are in control of what is happening, and it reduces the feeling that you are invading their space and doing something offensive or sexual to them.

If you take it easy and slow, you will make them comfortable and confident in what you are doing. You will preserve their respect and dignity. You will empower the remaining authority they still possess in their brain. You will enable them to feel like their life and opinion still does matter.

Protect identity, protect dignity, and protect reasonable rights
"Our lives begin to end the day we become silent about things that matter." – Martin Luther King Jr.

No matter where we live and under what generation, there are certain rights we want and demand as humans. We are creatures that require sustenance. We want and need to eat and drink. It is woven into our existence. Also, from birth, we have a longing and desire to connect. Over time, that feeling may develop into something else. But at the core, we desire to connect. We all have a natural desire to feel good, emotionally and physically. There is nothing like watching a happy baby interacting with their environment. Over time, based on how those rights and needs are fulfilled, it goes into shaping our identity, the very thing that produces our character, and the very thing that says who we are. We also learn our personal differences of right and wrong based on a universal standard of what right and wrong is. In our minds, we have a concept of right and wrong and we have governing thoughts that drive our actions and beliefs. Why am I bringing all of this up? Well, we have to understand that each of us has an ingrained identity. It is ours, and we do not want other to come and take it away from us.

Inside a person battling with memory loss is woven a natural fight to keep their identity. If we are a singer, writer, poet, engineer, parent, child or whatever our lot in life may be, we will do our very best to protect the integrity of that. It is important to a caregiver to plan to preserve that dignity that your loved one so cherishes.

What I found when addressing guardianship of my sister was that no matter how bad off she was, she still had rights that the courts required to be protected and addressed.   I had to have a high level of accountability for practically anything that was related to her. The court asked me on many occasions if I asked my sister permission regarding what she felt on the matter of finances, asset management, and health issues. What we were required to do in court is a minor reflection of what they are feeling. I cannot emphasize enough that you have to place it at the forefront of how you provide care. This will enable you to work in a cooperative spirit.

Sensitive areas of the body

"Sensitive people suffer more, but they love more and dream more." – Augusto Cury

Earlier I brought up how you should approach someone's personal space. In addition to that, you have to make yourself aware that there are a series of sensitive areas on their body that, because of the changes in their brain, will be especially sensitive. Because of the tension in my sister's body, due to the Lewy Bodies Dementia (LBD), she was hypersensitive to touches all over, mostly in areas of her major muscle groups.   Those areas were her arms, legs, back and abdominal area. When a LDB patient gets to the later stages of the disease, many lose their ability to communicate   verbally,   and   they   resort   to communicating   via   touch,   eye   movement,   facial expressions, and gestures. When it comes to touch, it was very interesting watching how my sister would react to it. She had a certain way of interpreting what was a rushed and intrusive gesture, versus a soft and respecting touch. I noticed that she needed all of her touches to be gentle for her not to interpret it as being a threat or causing some pain to her.

Because her taste for food had adjusted, the sensitivity of her lips and the skin surrounding her face also changed. It had become very sensitive to any touch. That area of skin would dry out a lot, so it required a lot of lotions in order to bring her comfort. Whenever I needed to communicate with her, I would have to take her hand and gently rub my fingers under her palm to get her to react to anything I needed to say to her. This became extremely important when it came to her losing the understanding of who I was. By doing this act, it helped spark her memory enough so she could identify who she was as well as who I was to her. Overall, it pays to stay observant to how they feel as well as how they feel when it comes to how they are touched.

❖Chapter 12 - Communication❖

Chapter 13 - Behavior Modification

"Human behavior flows from three main sources: desire, emotion, and knowledge." – Plato

When it comes to caring for your loved one, you will see some things surface that will be downright childish. They will do and say things that are off base and not so socially acceptable. You will even have instances where they will perform acts that resemble that of a child throwing a tantrum. However, as you go through this section, I want you to understand that you get to set the framework for how much of it will play out, and you also get to walk into this with your eyes open so you can take the right level of response so as not to bring harm to them or to yourself. What I want see grow within you from this chapter is a level of confidence that declares that you can manage this.

Do not use medication to fix

"Change your thoughts and you can change your world." - Unknown

Let me first state that I have a high respect for those in the medical field. Because of their training, they are getting exposed to a plethora of diseases, sicknesses, and bodily malfunctions, as well as mental and brain disorders. Doctors are taught to identify the ailment and prescribe treatment. In most cases, the prescription is in the form of medication. Globally, we as citizens of this world willfully accept what doctors say as gospel and ingest whatever they prescribe, based on their level of knowledge and treatment. There are also doctors who take the holistic and therapeutic approach. They spend a little more time with the patient and examine not just the symptoms but they look at lifestyle cause and effect. Let us say that a patient has accelerated heart rate. Instead of rushing to get the patient on some blood pressure meds, the doctor finds out through good questions what is triggering the event. Then, if they are in a non-critical position, they could talk about active strategies they could use to address it, such as reducing the sodium intake, and eating more fresh vegetables and drinking more water. They could also stay away from stressful people and situations for a while until they see a noticeable difference. They could do this along with prescribing the medication and give the patient an alternative to how they would want to address the issue, based on where they are with their will power and assistance. But what I am getting at is you need to try to address as many of your life's problems with behavioral modification versus medication. That way you can make empowered and informed choices to address the main symptoms.

With memory loss, the leading medication they prescribe has a success rate of about a year that it is effective. The other side effects such as mood swings, sleep disorder, anxiety, etc., are best controlled through a therapeutic approach, and use the medication as a gradual backup. You must understand that for most cases of dementia, it is irreversible and that over time, it will lead to brain death. As a caregiver, the medication will only give a limited quality of life. I want you to have a clear understanding of what your goals are and how you are going to approach how you are going to deal with them.

Coconut oil

***"The best doctors give the least medicines." –
Benjamin Franklin***

Since there is no cure on the market and being that people are getting fed up with not having any answers to how to address this dilemma, people have been pursuing all sorts of help, cures, and therapy. The danger is that there is some great help out there that are producing some health qualities, but I want to be clear, there has not been anything produced that has stopped or reversed the disease.

Now with that said, I do not want you to give up hope and stop seeking help and a cure. It is my aim and my fight to stay in this battle until every medical research company, legislation, pharmaceutical, medical, and government agency joins the fight in finding a cure. There are people who need relief and who needs their lives back. With all the non-pharmaceutical help out there, one interesting thing I found was the healing power of coconut oil. This is a substance that has multiple uses. It can be used internally and externally. It can be applied to the skin because it has soothing healing property for restoring moisture to the skin surface. Additionally, the University of Oxford has also found benefits of ingesting coconut oil and cooking with it. Such benefits include:

• Improving the body's use of insulin
• Improving cholesterol by increasing HDL (good cholesterol)
• Boosting thyroid function resulting in increased energy

- Acting as an antioxidant and natural antibiotic
- Improving overall health of skin and hair

Now, I do not what you to chuck your medicines and look at this as an end all cure. There still has not been enough research done on this, but it can be used in conjunction with the medication to help sustain the quality of life. But you can trust that I will stay on top of the research, so keep tuned into *CourageousCaregiver.org* and I will do my level best to make sure you get the latest information.

Aromatherapy

"Life is not measured by the number of breaths we take, but by the moments that take our breath away." – Maya Angelou

Who loves the smell of lilacs or daffodils? How about the smell of roses? What about the smell of your favorite cologne or perfume? When you think of those scents, they conjure up many memories. The smells tie you to a place and a time. The smells anchor your memory to key events that have happened in your life. So, I am recommending that you take advantage of positive smells. Take some time and experiment with various fragrances. The sense of smell will still be there for your loved one, but the way they interpret those memories may be a little twisted. Play around with subtle smells of sprays and candles. You can also use diffusers and melted wax. The smells will help improve the overall cognitive ability and it will also help improve the smell of the environment, which will help increase how pleasant people will feel for the experience.

Music

"Music can cure things that medications never will." – Unknown

This was one of my favorite tools in my arsenal. I know that I talked about this before, but I cannot emphasize how powerful it is. As the brain decreases in function, and it reduces to its most primitive state, you will see that music is an awesome equalizer. Music moves people. Music helps us remember who we are and what we are here for. Music makes us laugh and cry. It helps us think about the people we love. Music helps us think about what and whom we believe in. I have heard the phrase, "money makes the world go round." But, I also heard that "music is the rhythm that the world turns to."

Music has been said to have the power to calm the savage beast. With my little 5-month-old granddaughter, I would use music to calm and distract her. When she would throw her tantrums and get angry, I would take out my phone and turn on my Pandora station. I would play some of the old classics and it would get her attention. I would then pick her up and dance to song by Frank Sinatra and Michael Bublé. She will probably grow up liking that type of music because of the seeds that I have been planting in her little mind. But the music has a lot of cutting power to give her mind rest and realign her focus.

The same method that I would use on the young, I also applied to my older sister. My sister loved the R&B music from the 70s and 80's as well as gospel music from that era. So I would play it on the radio or on Pandora as much as possible. My sister would get in a more relaxed state of mind that made her easier to work with and relate to. The music took her to a place in time where she was in her prime and felt at her best. As the music played, she had a sense of comfort and joy.

I want you to think about when your loved ones were in their late teen years all the way up to the age of 30. Think about what music was popular during that time. Ask questions of their friends and family that knew them back then and then try to collect that type of music and have it ready and on hand. If your loved one seems tense, start off playing that music at a soft low level. Play around with the genre. You may also want to venture off into new music for them; I like the jazz station and, believe it or not, the classical. That is something that is simple and subtle, and you can play it at any volume level and each volume level has a different effect on the hearer. I hope this gives you a deeper level of confidence. Feel free to use this and look forward to the results you will be able to achieve.

Dance therapy
"Life is not about waiting for the storm to pass; it is about learning to dance in the rain." – Unknown

If your loved one is between level 0 to level 3, they will still have the mobility and dexterity that will enable them to move. Dancing is a wonderful way to move. But do not let them dance alone. Dance with them. Dance is a wonderful way to exercise and it is a powerful way to relate and connect. Crank up the music and have fun.

What if they say they cannot dance? So what? Just get up and move, laugh and have fun. Build healthy routines and beautiful memories that you can use to store up in your heart for when the hard times come.

I would not recommend getting into a style of dance that would cause or force them to learn anything new or complicated. Concentrate on one the movement and one activity. The cardiovascular exercise will prove to be valuable for increasing oxygenated blood flow the brain. So, relax, and feel free to boggy, shake, glide, smile, and have some fun.

Animal therapy

"Any glimpse into the life of an animal quickens our own and makes it so much the larger and better in every way." – John Muir

It is awesome to see the effect that animals have on soldiers that are struggling with PTSD. It pains me when I watch a fellow vet struggle with emotional trauma and pain for what war has caused in their body and mind. The sacrifice they make is huge, but it does not seem fair that they must also bear the mental trauma. I have a few friends that have taken on service dogs that are trained to sense when a vet's stress level was rising high, and the animals would calm the vet with a simple cuddle. It is powerful and earth changing what this therapy is doing, but it has a very similar and calming effect on dementia patients who are struggling with stress issues. Bear in mind that there might be some allergy issues, but if there is no problem look into leasing service from your local service animal group so they can periodically bring by an animal for therapy's sake.

Chapter 14 - Stress Management

"If the facts don't fit the theory, change the facts." – Albert Einstein

While I had the pleasure of talking to and getting to hear many different stories of dealing with dementia, one thing that was so common and apparent was that almost everyone was plagued with stress. The stress impacted the caregiver's personal health and mental state. It impacted relationships that they have with their loved one as well as others that they are involved with, be it family or friends. The stress impacted their work and productivity. Many have described it as being out in the middle of the ocean and treading water with no help or land for miles. They struggle to stay afloat. They worry if they will ever survive or if help will ever come. In this section, I want to offer some practical help and tips that I have used and that I have shared with others. I am sure as you read this it will trigger other things that you have learned. But this will prove to be a helpful reminder.

Personal care

"Do something today that your future self will thank you for." - Unknown

This is going to be hard for those of you who have gotten too emotionally attached. And as I am saying this, some of you will not be in a position where you can see the importance of this. You may be saying that there is no time for personal care. You might that your wife or husband, your mom or dad, or your sister or brother needs your full attention. The emotional draw is heavy and much of it comes from guilt. Some feel guilty because they think they are abandoning their loved one by taking time for themselves. However, as we neglect ourselves, we also take away from the quality of care that we can realistically provide. We also lose our objectivity, which helps us to see what quality care actually *is*. You have to make it a priority to provide personal care for yourselves and really take time to get a good picture of what that looks like. Let us explore some common options.

The power of a smile

"Every time you smile at someone it is an action of love, a gift to that person, a beautiful thing. – Mother Teresa

Smiling is to the brain as cardiovascular exercise is to the heart. A cardio workout promotes good blood flow and oxygen to the heart and brain and makes the heart muscles stronger and allows for it to withstand more. On the same level, as we smile or are in situations where we laugh and feel good, there is an enhancement of the flow of energy through the synaptic nerves. As we smile, we relax easier when faced with a tense situation. As we smile, we impact our spiritual ability to hope more above present situations. Our smiling can brighten our horizon of how we look at and choose to address life's situations. So exercise your right and power to turn up your smile. Take five minutes every morning and look in the mirror and just smile. Practice this for a week and then examine how you feel and how you handle the regular hassles of the day. If my guess is right, there will be some noticeable improvement in how you feel.

Rest

"Sleep is the golden chain that binds health and our bodies together." - Thomas Dekker

Serotonin is a hormone that is manufactured by your brain. This hormone controls how we handle obsessions and compulsions as well as anxiety. It is released when we rest. It is the brain's way of repairing itself from the daily grind of life. However, if we are on the edge all the time, our brains are not getting that opportunity to reset itself.

Put the blame on someone else

"Sometimes the easiest way to solve the problem is to stop participating in the problem." – Jonathan Mead

What I am going to suggest to you in this case seems shady and underhanded, but by using this, you will have peace of mind and the upper hand in managing a healthy and relational level of care with for the person that you love. Say your loved one have been adamantly engaging in practices that may be putting them at risk of harming themselves or others. And, let us also say, you have already approached them and asked as nice as possible, for them to stop what they have been doing, and you have yet only to receive anything but resistance, frustrations, and accusation. Your loved one may say, "You are not the boss of me. I don't have to do what you say. I am an adult and I know what's going on and I can make my own decision." They are saying this while trying to stick a knife into a toaster or drive a car on the wrong side of the road, with you or even small kids in the car with them. Seems scary, however, this happens more times than not when trying to get your independent loved one to step back and step down from engaging in risky activity.

Now, before you get to the state of having to use other authority figures, you may want to explore the reasons they have for doing the task that may be putting them at risk. People want to feel validated. Ask them why they feel so strongly about the thing that they are doing. Work with them to think of alternatives to what they are doing. You want to do this before you start insisting they make a change. Make them feel that they are a part of the decision-making process.

You love them and really wish that they would heed your warning and cooperate and stop. What should be simple becomes an emotional struggle and a match of wills. What seems logical and right now becomes a battle for identity. They might say something like, "I have always done it this way, and I will keep on doing this way." This is a powerful and painful statement on their part. I would first of all suggest, when emotions run high, to deliberately step back. Do not try to one-up and win an argument. That technique does not work. The logic center of the brain is one of the first things to go. Plus, you do not want to stay in confrontation mode with a person with dementia, simply because the emotion tied to the event you want them to change can be engrained, and they will associate you with tension in their life. So you will need to consider using scapegoats. I prefer using authorities of higher powers.

For example, one issue could be if they were prone to walking away. Think of someone with authority that they would respect and use them as a voice and a reason to modify their behavior. You could say that the police just sent out a notice that there were people mugging older people in the neighborhood. That way, they would have the police to blame and a potential threat to the neighborhood and a reason to not walk off alone. Is it a lie? It just may be, but it is also so close to the truth, that they may not question it. At the heart of the matter, you want to avoid pushback while setting up good safety parameters.

This can be applied to practically every issue you are facing, such as in the area of bathing. If they hate washing up, create a reason for them to wash that would seem important, such as them seeing an old family friend in a special place. That event may not be true and meeting may not be real, but you can get them cleaned and dressed and then go do something and make it seem special. If they were refusing to take medication, before yelling at them or trying to force it on them, you want to first consider the alternatives. What is the medication and how is it affecting them? Are they getting any positive results from the meds? Are the pills too big and hard to swallow? Could it be administered in another, less intimidating form? Perhaps after reviewing all the other concerns and options and helping them understand the option, you find they are still giving you resistance. Indicate to them that without this medication, they will need to go to the hospital and the doctors may need to give the medication to them through an injection. End with an alternate choice that may be meaningful and persuasive to encourage them to go the easier route.

The power of journaling
"Journaling and writing your thoughts down every day is a great way to make sure you choose your life more than others do" – Unknown

Personally, I am not a fan of journaling. I hate writing, (yet I find myself writing this book). I am not the type who likes to get in touch with my feelings. At first, I had to force myself to think about something I could put into writing. Once I thought about it, I had to ask myself why I needed to write it. When it comes to the thought process, we have a variety of random thought that fly through our heads within a fraction of a minute. However, at the rate we think, it is very difficult and disorganizing to try to function just off of a random thought. A person who does this will find it difficult to get things done.

Journaling helps to get the mind, body and spirit in sync, so they can work together to accomplish the common goal. There are various reasons why you should journal. You can write about your highs and lows. You can write about some lessons learned, or you can write about some plan or task that you would like to accomplish. Even if you do not accomplish it or decide to go to a new plan, the journal gives you a good point of reference that shows you how much you have changed or evolved as a person. Journaling helps you see and navigate around the chaos of life.

Join the fantasy

"Fantasy is hardly a way of escaping reality... It's a way of understanding it." – Lloyd Alexander

I have been accused of messing with people's heads. I have this ability to listen to people, and if I feel that the conversation is getting boring, I can ask questions or make comments to add color to it to make it a bit more exciting to my taste. I developed this skill from trying to deal with my sister when she would have deep moments of frustration. There were times when she would talk and not make any rational sense whatsoever. She would try to recall events that I knew she did not have her facts straight on, and every time I would try to correct her all it would do was set her off.

I found that the less I would fight with her, and the less I would try to correct her memory, the better I felt. I did not want to find myself in constant battles with her because it raised both of our stress levels. The stress was causing dissension between us, and it was impacting my health. I had to consciously choose to let it go. I had to let go of being right. I had to let go of winning the battles. I had to come to terms with the fact that my sister's brain was not going to be healthy, but was gradually getting worse. Her reality was not going to be the same that I had. And I had to be completely okay with this.

What worked best for me was to reduce my level of communication down to childlike elementary speaking. The conversations would sound silly to an outsider, but for us, it was an atmosphere of peace. I set a goal for my sister and I to have as much fun as we could together. So I would listen to her, and I would embellish on her facts and try to make them funny for her.

This next part will seem a little mean, but every day I would take my sister to and from her adult daycare. At that time, my transportation was not reliable. My vehicle gas gauge was broken, and I would periodically run out of gas and not know it. She would make comments about me running out of gas and this would worry her a bit. This stuck with her, so she would bring it up all the time. Instead of letting it annoy me, I would tell her that I kept a harness in the back, and if we happened to run out of gas, I would hitch her to the car and let her pull us to the nearest gas station. This conversation would happen every day. And the response would be the same. She would give me a look of shock, and say she would not be performing that task. She would then think about what was just said, and then begin to laugh after visualizing how silly that would look. My humor with her made her feel respected and it kept our bond strong and refreshing. I encourage you to please take time to have some fun and try not to be all about the business and mechanics of taking care of your loved one. Life is to be lived and you do not want to miss it.

Balanced love

"Life is like riding a bicycle. To keep your balance, you must keep moving." – Albert Einstein

I know you really care about your loved one, or else you would not have read this far into this book. I know that some of what I am saying is resonating with you. You understand the gravity of what you are facing, and you care at a deep level and have made sacrifices in order to provide care. For those of you engaged in direct care, I commend you. For those of you who are learning how to maintain your spirit and grow during this process, I can clearly say, you are super human.

It takes a mature spirit to see that there is a balance that must exist between caring for your loved one and caring for yourself. The expression and passion of love can drive you to do some extraordinary things, and it can also force you to define love in a way that could be outside of your healthy norm of living. An example of this would be a woman who is in a physically abusive relationship, who in her heart really loves her husband, and even hears those words coming from her spouse in between the beatings he issues.   To an outsider, this is wrong and something must be done about it. You might wonder why does she not just run away or tell someone. To her, it is not that simple. It is not cut and dry. There are deeply wrapped emotions and a bond that is not easily broken.

I am not saying that caring for a loved one under extreme circumstances is abusive, but what I am saying is that a caregiver can push themselves into a blind frenzy and not see some unhealthy patterns developing as they provide care. Some do not stop to take a health assessment to look at their own vital signs. Rest is put to a minimum. Eating healthy becomes a secondary thought. Stress runs high and very little breaks are scheduled in order to decompress. There are aches and pains that are being ignored. What about a vacation? When was the last time one was taken? How about assessing how you currently feel about your loved one. On a scale from 1 to 10, where 10 is the high, how much do you really love the person you are caring for? If you are in need of help and support, are you reaching out to the local or on-line support groups?

Love for self, has to take a high priority; a much higher priority over the person you are caring for. You have to develop a snapshot of what that looks like and then function in that parameter. You have to draw healthy boundaries of what you can and cannot do and then stick to it. On areas where you cannot help, you must seek out others. This is a sign of strength and maturity and not a sign of failure or weakness. You owe it to yourself to take care of yourself.

Suicide risk

"Until you are broken, you don't know what you're made of. It gives you the ability to build yourself all over again, but stronger than ever." - *Unknown*

Emotions can run high for caregivers. Facing dementia can be very overwhelming. Especially as you see the progression of the disease, or after you have been berated by the person you love well after you poured out your heart, soul, and energy to provide quality care. It is painful, and it cuts deep. After someone experiences so much abuse, a person can reach a breaking point. Sometimes, a person will start to get so discouraged that they become hopeless and doubtful about the future. They may even get to the point where they want no part of where the future may lead. The emotional pain becomes so great that they see no way out.

If you are a caregiver, and you are struggling with these emotion, I ask that you put this book down, and go call a friend and let them know how you feel. Your friend may not have the right answers to what you are going through or what you are feeling, but I can assure you, the weight of what you are feeling is too heavy to bear alone. If you have thoughts about hurting yourself, and the thoughts are becoming more frequent, you may need to step back for a moment and reassess your level of care you are providing. If you are feeling that low and depressed over what you are experiencing, there is no shame in reaching out for help. You do yourself nor your loved one no justice by allowing yourself to stay stressed out over what you are facing. Take time out, call someone, and seek out help. If you are reading this book on behalf of someone else who is a caregiver, call them and let them know that you are there for them. We have to hold each other up during these trying times. If things get too overwhelming, call 911 or your doctor, or call your local suicide hotline. There are people committed and dedicated to helping you.

Homicide risk

"Hatred paralyzes life; love releases it. Hatred confuses life; love harmonizes it. Hatred darkens life; love illuminates it." -Martin Luther King Jr.

It is extremely frustrating to help someone who seems resentful or comes off as abrasive. People with dementia can have some very heavy mood swings where they will become rude, insulting, and combative. These acts can become hostile and threatening to the point that you are forced to get physical with them. You may even feel as if you *want* to get physical with them in order to get them under control. There is a definite homicide risk when it comes to giving someone such intense care.

Trust me when I say that if you are driven to that point, and if you take the next step, it is a no way out situation. Once you are pondering those emotions in your heart, it does not take much to push you to the next level. The next level could really hurt your loved one. Let us think about that for a moment. This is a person you love. A person you chose to step up for, and lay down your life for, and care for. You may be the only person in their life that really cares. But you let circumstances get so extreme that you feel like you are watching a movie of your life and you are the villain. You might even ask yourself how things could have gotten that bad.

Before you say another word to your loved one, I ask that you stop! Assess the patterns and the tension. You picked up this book because you needed help. I am here for you. I know what you are feeling. I have been there myself. If things are desperate, go to my website and shoot me a message. I will respond. But I sincerely ask you to back away from the thought you are having. Seek out help. Find someone to talk to. You do not want to let your rage run so high that you reach out and hurt the one you have committed to care for.   The thoughts and actions come with a weight of regret that you cannot get rid of. If your rage is running high, now is the time to think about some rapid changes you have to make in how care is provide. Seek out other relatives that may be willing to help or that can assist and take a load off.   Take a breather from all that you have been doing. I highly recommend that you seek out a wellness coach, so they can help you navigate through these rough waters.   After all, you started caring for your loved one because you wanted them to be safe and healthy. So why would you allow yourself to be the unhealthiest thing around them? Pick up the phone and ask for help.   There is more help out there than you know.

Relaxation and personal cardio

"Remember the feeling you get from a good run is far better that the feeling you get from sitting around wishing you were running." – Sarah Condor

For me, this is my favorite thing to do. I get so charged when I engage in a cardio activity. There is something about moving and grooving at a pace where you are huffing a puffing and pushing your body to a higher level. I like walking on our local nature trails or going to our local mall and doing laps. When I exercise, I push myself to the point where I breathe with effort. My heart beats faster, but the best side effect of all is that it pushes oxygenated blood to my brain and clears my head. I feel like I get more refined and creative thoughts when engaged in physical activity. So, if you are stressed, take a 20-minute break and walk. If you cannot go out and walk, then you can at least walk in place. It may look silly to others, but it will do wonders for bringing down your stress level.

Also, as a caregiver, you work hard at creating a safe and comfortable environment for your loved one where they can rest and be at peace. However, I am more so interested in you taking time for yourself to really rest and unwind. You owe it to yourself to get between six and eight hours of sleep a night. If your loved one is exhibiting behavior issues that may come into conflict with you resting, such as roaming the house at night or leaving, then I would suggest sleeping in shifts with someone else who can care for your loved one. If that does not work, and if you have a person who likes to sneak out of the house while you are sleeping, then you may want to change the locking system to make it a bit more difficult to exit the doors.

I have seen some families where the loved one would eat at night and consume all the food that was in the home while the others are sleep. Some families have had to go as far as child-proofing their home to the point of locking down areas where they do not want their loved ones to roam. This at least gives a deeper level of peace of mind, which will enable you as a caregiver a chance to rest.

264 ❖ Courageous Caregiver

Overall, take the time to assess if you are getting rest and exercise, and if you are not, really look at the reason as to why it is not happening. Creatively think about what can be changed in order for those healthy qualities to be implemented. If there is an overwhelming matter that is preventing you from getting rest, then you owe it to yourself to seek out help. And as a last resort, you will want to consider assisted living or a nursing home for your loved one. Overall, you have to take care of yourself, or you will not be in position to take care of anyone else.

Love with detachment and boundaries
"Detachment is not that you should own nothing, but that nothing should own you." – Ali ibn abi Talib

"I love you so much, it hurts." This is a common phrase when you have a relationship going through its trials of peaks and valleys. Pain is an awesome teacher. It keeps us awake at night and moves us in our level of thought of who we are and how we will live the lives we have. We sometimes get this misconception that if we love a little more that it can smooth out and resolve all of our problems. However, love can be blinding and draw us close to the flames.

In order for love to thrive, the feeling has to be mutual in expression. However, what does it take to love a person who has lost their capacity to reciprocate, let alone, express any form of gratitude or respect? If you are tasked with being a caregiver, this can be really hard for you to take. In order for you to feel whole, you have to declare your personal boundaries and limitation for which you can take. You have to make it clear and understood what you will and will not take. I will use

❖Chapter 14 - Stress Management❖

the example of profanity. A person with dementia will resort to primal expression and can be easily triggered by using foul language. Therefore, clear boundaries have to be expressed so they can develop some form of internal messaging that they have to try to control their expressions. As you mature as a caregiver with your knowledge and strategies to help them curb their foul mouth, along with declaring boundaries, you stand a winning chance of walking away with your sanity. The other thing with boundaries is knowing your limitation and pre-determining the healthiest response to things that cross the line. By establishing a pre-determined response, it gives you empowerment and control over the situation versus the events controlling the outcome. What I am trying to direct you to do here is develop an objective strategy that will enable you to step back and assess what is happening before reacting to things. This equips you with the emotional tools to still love but to do the right thing based on a criteria of overall health based on the facts and events that are being presented to you at a given time.

Wellness coach
"Coaching is the universal language of change and learning." – CNN

It is hard to admit when you are over your head and need help. Trust me. I have been there. I am the first to admit that I am full of pride and will fight tooth and nail to do something by myself before asking for help, even to the point of it almost killing me. That attitude has led me into a lot of scrapes where I literally almost lost my life. It takes a bigger man to rise and say he needs help. As I have matured, I began to see that there is nothing wrong with getting a little help.

One area that people secretly struggle with is their emotions. Sometimes the things that we think about frighten us, and we have to take a step back to assess what we are experiencing. Even in our assessment, we can find that some of the thoughts are tangled, dark, and overwhelming. When caring for someone who is getting progressively worse, it is easy to feel helpless and hopeless. It can become very difficult to even express yourself.

In my struggle with caring for my sister, I found myself blessed with help from some really good professionals. The counselors I ran into allowed me to express myself while not making me feel guilty or bad in any kind of way for what I felt. A good counselor will help validate your feelings and help you identify where they are coming from. In addition, they will help you identify triggers of anxiety and then will work with you to develop a winning strategy that will help you feel empowered and equip you to face your feelings and interpret the facts in a healthy way. Once I was able to get help with my thoughts and anxiety, I was then able to objectively see where I was causing some of my own problems as well as where I could get additional help to face some of the struggles I was having.

My advice to you, if you are overwhelmed and you have no one to turn to, is to try to seek out good counsel.   I recommend calling the Alzheimer's Association and seeing if they can direct you to some resources. Next, I would direct you to talk to your family doctor and see if they have any recommendations. You could also talk to your local religious leaders and see if they can direct you to anyone in your area that has experience with what you are going through. I will do my very best with trying to keep my finger on the pulse of this matter and try to keep my website up to date with people who may be of service to you. But do not give up hope. We are all here for each other.

Massage

"Take care of your body. It is the only place you have to live in." – Unknown

I have never had one of these, professionally, but I have heard some amazing things about them. So I had to throw this into the book. I work out on occasion, and I know that there are times when I push myself to an extreme, where the results are some really sore muscles. And I think to myself, a massage would really feel wonderful.

This is one way that you can take time out to simply pamper yourself. There are some reputable places where you can go, and you will find that the atmosphere is designed to bring you into a deep relaxing state of mind a body. If you have been going at it and pushing your body to the max, I am pleading with you, add this to your immediate things to do—relieve stress and take a load off.

Hugs

"Hugs were invented to let people know you love them without having to say anything." – Unknown

Hugs are one of the best ways to express love and care for others as well as for you. They are therapeutic. A hug says so much, without saying anything. As you give hugs, you also receive them. They are so liberating and powerful. I feel sorry for the people who declare that they do not do hugs. They are missing out on one of the most powerful sparks of life.

Growing up, my parents were not that affectionate to me. I do not recall too many hugs ever coming from my parents, unless it was on special occasions. When I reached my teen years, I was a very closed-off type of person. I hated hugs because I did not know how to respond to it when people tried to give them to me. Later, as an adult, I went into the military. The US Marine Corps was not exactly hug-friendly. So I was comfortable and felt at home there. It was not until I met my wife that I transitioned into a hugger. Her family was very affectionate and loving. The hugs I got were so refreshing and empowering, and I liked it.

These days, I hug practically everyone I meet, friends and strangers. I am very adamant about making people feel like they matter and that no matter what society says about living a closed off sheltered life, I do not have to function that way. Usually, I limit myself to not hugging at work. Most workplaces frown on that type of connection and so I only do it if invited to.

But for therapeutic sake, be free and choose to connect. Hug your loved one. Hug your spouse, children, parents, family, and friends. There is a release of endorphins that occurs that reduces stress as you engage in a hug. So open up wide and break out beyond your barriers and hug somebody. It just may save your life.

Avoiding burnout

"What lies behind us and what lies before us are tiny matters compared to what lies within us." – Ralph Waldo Emerson

First of all, I would say in order to know what burnout is, I have to present a point of reference. If you have ever lifted weights, you know that the goal is controlled repetition. Pushing beyond your perceived limitations. You know you hit a point of muscle fatigue when you think that you cannot push it any further. But then, you find just enough in you to do one more rep. You feel that burn and you want to quit, but something is pushing you to go forward. With any good muscular train routine, you have to alternate the muscle training day so you can give your muscles time to heal and enable you to work out on the next cycle.

Where burnout comes into play is when you are not listening to the events that are playing in your life. You are getting up every day and pushing beyond your limit, but you have not set a standard of where you will stop, nor have you put into schedule where you will rest and reset. Without this, you will have a life that is out of balance. In order to avoid burnout, you have to be aware that it is happening. In order to do that, you have to take time to assess how you feel. You have to ask: at what times of the day am I getting adequate rest? How much has my life changed since I started providing direct care? Do I spend any time doing anything of leisure that I really like? How well do I know myself in the sense that I know what relaxation really means to me and not a modified definition based on my given circumstance? Do I ask for and allow others to help? These are just a few questions to consider when getting things started. I am sure as you address these questions, you will be able to come up with deeper questions that can move you to an area in your life that will keep you from burning out.

Either way, you are not a machine. You are a person with a life and with feelings. Do not let the disease or your compassion rob you of a portion of precious life that you need to live. I understand that you have been called to make a great sacrifice on behalf of the person you love, and just like any good soldier that has gone to war, you have stepped up and put up a good fight. And like any good soldier, you are obligated and mandated to take R&R—rest and relaxation. So mold that into your schedule and breathe a little.

Alcohol and drug escape

"Running away from any problem only increases the distance from the solution. The easiest way to escape from the problem is to solve It." – Unknown

There is nothing wrong with wanting to escape from some of the pressures you are facing. Stresses in life pop up all the time, no matter what you are facing. People have a variety of ways they choose to decompress. I feel that, and I deeply understand. I have worked some very crappy jobs in my past and some of them I came close to losing my life on the job. The stress from the near misses alone was enough to make me take a few days off, or even want to take a stiff drink.

Now, do not get me wrong. I am not slamming drinking, but I am warning against using alcohol or drugs as a means to address your stress. Both have a high potential of impairment. Taking care of a loved one or even yourself while impaired is dangerous. I am sure you have heard it before, so I am not trying to repeat the same song. But I am trying to help you understand that you have to plan ahead that there will be stress, and you have to plan ahead on how to best deal with your stresses before you get deep into them. My goal is to empower you and to increase your limit of choices. The more choices you have, the better outcome you can implement.

Some of the things that I have implemented were going for walks and talking to a friend that understands. Try getting a sitter and do a day or night out. If you love music, find some that will uplift you. If you are into arts and craft, paint a masterpiece. Go on a date. Go to the pet shop and love on some animals. You make your list and do what better suits you, depending on your level of stress.

But I clearly know that alcohol or drugs as a means to deal with stress will rob you of things that you cannot get back. They have risks of sending you down a dark hole that you may not ascent. You will create dependencies that you will become powerless to let go. My passion is to bring health back into your life. We are kindred spirits, and we share the same passion. We love our loved one, and we want to feel love for ourselves. I am begging you that if you are in this situation, be bold enough to stop. Stop before it is too late.

Sleep management
"If you correct your mind, the rest of your life will fall into place." – Lao Tzu

I love sleep. I love it in the morning; I love it at night. I love it anytime I can get it. It makes it all right.

It feels so good and refreshing. I have hated it, ever since I was a kid, when people would come along and choose to disturb my sleep. My sleep was bought at a high price and I cannot let those sacrifices happen in vein. Soldiers are hunkered down, in a lookout position in some third world country, defending my country, over there, so I can sleep in peace every night. Thanks for your sacrifice, my brothers and sisters in arms.

Sleep is so important, and it is one of the things that a caregiver will quickly sacrifice for the sake of caring. It is a proven fact that a person who is lacking sleep functions as if they were impaired by alcohol. A lack of rest can also lead to rapid brain deterioration, due to stress and lack of oxygenated blood going to the brain. When we rest, this is the moment when our body repairs itself from the damages we have done to it from our day. Without sleep, we can promote an environment where we will fail to thrive, as well as open ourselves to mental disorders.

So what do we do about it? You have a loved one that is demanding or up at night, or one that is a flight risk. You have a loved one that is potentially violent. So, how can you get to a state where you can lay down and rest? First of all, you have to understand that your sleep and your loved one's sleep go hand in hand. About 20 percent who suffer with Dementia or Alzheimer's may develop Sundowning. This is where there is a mental confusion about night and day. Later in the day, more confusion, anxiety and stress develops, according to the Alzheimer's Association. This will impact their desire to sleep, along with some other medical conditions that may exist, such as restless leg syndrome, sleep apnea (where you at times, stop in your breathing pattern while sleep), incontinence, or urinary tract infection. Either way, whatever is affecting them, what I am going to share with you will prove to be valuable to help them, as well as yourself, get a wonderful night's sleep.

Schedule management

"You can do anything, but not everything." - David Allen

This is something that you have to evaluate and adjust in order to better manage your environment as well as any activity you allow to be packed into your day. Whether you are at home with them all day, or if you are with them part time, these minor schedule adjustments will help improve your resting outcome. As I explore the other sections you will see the importance of schedule adjustments.

Lighting

"Small lights have a way of being seen in a dark world." – Neil A. Maxwell

During the waking hours, and as often as possible throughout the day, you want the home and environment well lit. You want as much natural sunlight to be a part of the day, and in the evenings, you will want to make the lighting soft, yet bright. As bedtime approaches, reduce the lighting. You may want to install dimmer switches.

Comfortable sleeping environment

"Harmony makes small things grow, lack of it makes great things decay." – Socrates

You want the area where they sleep to be the most comfortable place on earth. The bedding should be simple and soft. Linen should be changed often (in the event of incontinence and bed wetting). The air should be fresh, but not overpowering. You can adjust this with aromatherapy fragrance plugins or fresh cut flowers. The room for your loved one should be free of clutter and trip hazards. I personally like to go to sleep to soft music. So I would invest in some form of music player that has a timer that can shut itself off. Either way, you want your loved one to identify this room as a place of comfort and relaxation. When they enter, they should be persuaded to get into a state of comfortable sleep. This would not be a bad idea for you to do the same to your own sleeping environment.

You will want to monitor and get feedback as to how they feel about climate control. Check to see if they are the type of person that likes to sleep where it is cool or warm. Do they like pillows and what type and how many? Do they sleep with a blanket, or comforter, or are they the type who likes to sleep with just a sheet? These are very important thing you will want to explore for maximum comfort. One other thing to make the zone comfortable is to make sure the doors and windows can be secured. For wanderers, you will want to invest indoor sensors and motion detectors, as well as set up limited access to areas that you will declare as a safe zone.

Meal times
"Let food be medicine and let thy medicine be food." – Hippocrates

This is one of those schedule things that I told you about. When it comes to our body performance, our eating content and schedule is core to 80% of what our body will experience. The average person eats three meals a day, and they throw in a snack here and there. What I recommend is that you pack your heaviest meals within your breakfast or lunch period. Here is where you give them energy based foods, such as fruits or sweeter items. This is where you give the carb based starches. Later in the day, you want dinner to be a light meal and you want it to be foods that are low carb and less energy based foods. You really want to avoid sweets and deserts at this meal. Also, you want to cut off eating at four hours before the expected bedtime.

Daily activity

"Don't mistake movement for achievement. It is easy to get faked out by being busy. The question is: 'Busy doing what?'' – Jim Rohn

You will have to be very deliberate about what you are going to pack into your loved one's day and when. My recommendation is that you plan for plenty of activities throughout the beginning of the day up through the afternoon. Try to keep them functioning and engaged with appointments and activities. After dinner, you can taper off the activity, and by doing so, you will have burned off their energy so they can be in a prime state to rest. Use dinner time as a way to slow the day down. Almost make it dull so that you will, in a way, bore them into wanting to go to sleep. They will have had a full, eventful, and fulfilling day, and they will be happy to rest. This will in turn, enable you to get a good night's rest.

Watch for triggers

"When you set yourself on fire, people will want to see you burn." – John Wesley

There are things that will cause your loved one to get emotionally ramped up. You must make yourself aware of those things and set limits on how they can invade your life. One such trigger could be the news. Many of the stories are hard, sad, and depressing. The news is not all that healthy to consume even if you have a healthy brain. Children are another factor. If you have a child with a lot of energy who may be a little loud and out of control, then you may want to consider other living arrangements for the child or your loved one if you expect them and yourself to get healthy sleep. Be careful of the volume of music and the type of music you are allowing to be played in your loved one's presence. During the day, I would suggest you play music with energy, but in the evenings, play music that is soft and calming.

Watch for the snap back

"If you cannot be positive, then at least be quiet." – Joel Osteen

This was a touchy one for me. When I am tired and trying to hide the fact that I am tired, I can give a verbal or even a non-verbal response that can be harsh and cutting. So, in order to combat this, I had to be deliberate about getting good sleep. My sleep and my loved one's sleep were interconnected. My sister could pick up on my body language and she could either know to back off or become anxious and respond in a not so pleasant manner. I had to learn to get myself under control.

Sleep aid
"At the end of the day, you can either focus on what's tearing you apart, or on what's holding you together."
- Unknown

As a last resort, if you cannot make adjustments that work, then talk to your loved one's doctor, as well as your, own and consider trying a sleep aid. Many other, highly skilled doctors, and I, will recommend using natural sleep aid before jumping into the heavier drugs. The leading brand in the market that you can get at any drug store or health food store is *melatonin*. It is simple and mild and has no after effect. Beyond that, seek the advice of your doctor if you need anything stronger to help you or your loved one.

Show up for your own life
"Don't wait for someone to bring you flowers. Plant your garden and decorate your soul." – **Unknown**

You are unique and there is no ne like you. You have gifts and talents that the world needs to experience. There is a voice in you, waiting to get out. There are lives that you were meant to impact. People you were made to love. Places you were called to go, see, and experience. There are things that you were meant to do. With this simple section, I am trying to tell you that if you are playing the martyr because you are engaging in care, stop it! You must not completely erase your life, hopes, and dreams simply because you chose to care for someone else. Caring may take time away from you fully experiencing your dreams, but do not let it take away from you working on your dreams, gifts, and talents. There is always something you can do. Find a way to fit something in your day, and just keep at it. If the Creator is willing and compassionate enough, He may grant you a wonderful opportunity to live out your dream, in spite of your circumstances, no matter what. Do not stop believing. Do not stop living. Do not stop loving simply because you chose to do a courageous thing by stepping up to care. But fight to show up for your own life.

You cannot go back, but you can be real and wisely move forward
"When you bring peace to your past, you can move forward to your future." – Unknown

I wish they could invent a time machine where I could go back and correct the mistakes I may have made. Or where I could stop myself from saying some things that should have never exited my mouth. Many wrongs come to mind that I wish I could have undone. I guess it is part of the divine design that we cannot go back. Some of the painful experiences that occurred in many people's lives were the very thing that moved them into the strong, wise, mature, caring compassionate people they are today. I used to regret my past and all the negative things that I experienced, but now I embrace it. It gives my life journey more color and relevance to my destination. I am far more appreciative of the good times, simply because I experienced the bad times.

I am sharing this with you so that you may be able to find relief and growth through your experience. I know that if you are caught up with the throws of this disease, it is easy to lose sight of your identity and where all of this is headed. In fact, I want to share with you this simple truth: the future possesses that which you show up with. If you chose to bring pain, sadness, misery, brokenness, and bitterness in with you, then that is what will be waiting for you in in the very near future. If you chose to walk with truth, love, hope, peace, patience, kindness, health, and wholeness, that is what will await you on your next turn.

You get to shape your change, and you are allowed to be the master of what the change will look like, simply by adjusting your choices and your reactions to circumstances. Be in the present with so much love that the future cannot help but return love in abundance to you once you get there.

It is not what you know, but how you apply what you know

"It's not hard to make decisions once you know what your values are." – Roy E. Disney

I am sure you are gaining a great deal of knowledge by reading this text. I thank you for sticking with me this far. You took the risk and bought this book, and I hope I have not failed you. I pray that I have taken your mind and your heart to a higher level of knowledge, love, and insight. To be honest, by the time you are done with this book, you may know as much, if not more, than many of the first year residents at many of the nation's hospitals. However, that does not qualify you to go off and open a practice. I hold high respect for those in the medical field. I have come across some really great practitioners. Some that are so knowledgeable in their fields and who could talk for hours and dazzle you with what they know.

However, it is crucial to know when to pull back or even limit how much they know. There are things that doctors know, about certain ailments, that if they chose to give us all of the information, we would cease to have hope, due to the information overload. A good doctor knows that they are required to tap into a person's hope and belief system to aid them in their own personal health. A doctor has to have a great bedside manner, which promotes health and hope. A doctor must give an impression, whenever they can, that the patient will get or feel better, simply for the fact that most doctors know that if a patient loses their will to live, then it will not take much to push them over the edge.

As a caregiver, it is equally important to screen what we say to our loved ones who are struggling with dementia. They have to see and feel that you are doing your very best to make their life and existence one of happiness and love. They must see how you are fighting for their health, so they can feel willing to let you come alongside them and aid them in establishing stability in their life. Take what you know and apply it with gentleness and compassion. Try not to come off as a know-it-all, but slowly and in small chunks share what you can, and apply the rest in practice in the safeguards you are setting up for them. But above all, do some good self-evaluation to make sure you are not coming off as condescending. They can sense that and may choose to fight or resist you in your process and plan to help them.

Cortisol level

"If I had nine hours to chop down a tree, I'd spend the first six sharpening my ax." – Abraham Lincoln

What is cortisol? This is an adrenal gland secretion that is produced in your body whenever faced with a stressful situation. It impacts glucose metabolism, blood sugar regulation, insulin release, immune function, and inflammation response. It is triggered by the situation when we are either going to fight or flight. When this happens, we could experience a sudden burst of energy, heightened memory function, increased immunity, or even lower sensitivity to pain. Cortisol is important to the body. However, if a person is not deliberate with practicing relaxation techniques, this could lead to impaired cognitive performance, suppressed thyroid function, blood sugar imbalance such as hyperglycemia, decreased bone density, decreased muscle tissue, high blood pressure, lowered immunity, high inflammation, and increased abdominal fat. I want to share with you some great relaxation techniques that have been proven to get some great results: guide imagery (visualization exercises); journaling, self-hypnosis or neurological linguistic programming (NLP); exercise; yoga; listening to music; deep breathing; meditation; affirmations. This is a short list, and I am sure there are many other things that you can try. But my point is that you must be deliberate to drive that stress away from you and fight for your good and balanced health.

Breathe

"That breath you just took... That's a gift." – Rob Bell

Breathing is something that we do naturally. Some of us have to struggle with it more than others. If we are still living, then we do this day in and day out. It is vital to our existence. However, in this section, I am not talking about normal breathing that we do just to survive. What I am talking about is a level of breathing that we do that keeps us focused and engaged with how we are breathing.

First of all, let us try a simple exercise. Breathe in for four counts and hold it for four counts, then breathe out for four counts, then hold it for four count, then allow yourself to breath normal. What I wanted you to notice is your chest, abdomen and diaphragm. Did you notice any tension in the muscles as you breathed? Next, I want you to try it again, but this time, I want to you to think about just letting go of the tension in your abdominal area. As you breathe in, let your stomach push out and do not try to resist or hold your stomach in. You will notice after breathing in and out for a few times that you will feel tension start to leave other parts of your body. As I mentioned above, it is important to control your cortisol levels, but it is also vital that you practice the easiest thing of all, breathing, and bring your stress level down to a state where you feel like you are calm and in charge of all of your faculties.

Be tuned into your patience

"Patience is not the ability to wait but how you act while you're waiting." – Joyce Meyer

In today's society, we are conditioned to be hyper busy and to multi-task. We talk to people and try to carry on multiple conversations at the same time. We could be face-to-face with one person, while talking to another on the phone, with our Bluetooth in our ear, and texting another person, while Facebook messaging another. All while driving a vehicle. Now if this is not a recipe for disaster, I do not know what is.   After thinking about this, I needed to take a breather. People, we need to fight to find a way to simplify life and slow some things down. Studies have shown that people can adapt to multitasking. However, their focus is greatly diminished.   Their ability to communicate effectively declines.   Listening skills drop 60% based on the number of communication elements that a person tries to maintain at once.

Now, take this into an environment where you are dealing with a person who is memory challenged. They have limited speaking capabilities as well as limited means of understanding verbal or situational nuances.   And if we find ourselves multitasking in communication with them, it can become very frustrating to them, and they will in turn make it frustrating to you. I have found that what works best is to pare down and focus on them when I am choosing to interact. I try to quiet the environment and put on soft music in the background before engaging in conversation.   This helps calm them and makes them more responsive to what is said. If they receive it better, they respond better and that in turn reduces any stresses that would normally pop up and it makes for a better overall communication situation.

Build a sanity sanctuary

"Within you there is a stillness and a sanctuary to which you can retreat any time." – Hermann Hesse

There is a line from the hit TV show *Cheers* that goes, "Some people want to go where everybody knows their name." This was a place of love, laughter, realness, and a place where you could relax and blow off stream.

We all need to do that at times. Taking care of a loved one is not easy. It takes a brave person with a strong spirit and heart full of love to this. I commend each of you for stepping up to this task. Just like Superman had his Fortress of Solitude and Batman had his Bat Cave, so you too need a place where you can steal away to, where you can regroup and collect your thoughts. You have to be very deliberate and fight for this. I have seen some who care to such an extreme, and they built their lifestyle in such a way, that they would never get a moment's rest away from their loved one. This method will not work for the long run and will lead to your personal demise. You have to choose to step back and take a break. I am not saying neglect your loved one. But what I am saying is to at least start with taking ten minutes out of each day that is just yours and that will be non-interrupted. Go to a place where you will not be disturbed. Turn of the phone and TV and unplug for a moment and try to soak up as much quiet time that you can get for yourself. Some are saying, at this time, that they really love the noise, music, and activity. They may be well and good, but what I am proposing is to try to see and evaluate the impact it may have on your brain, stress level, and outlook on things, to simply soak in about ten minutes of quiet time. If it works for you and you see some benefits, then try to carve out more. My point is, you owe it to yourself to take that break and find a place and time that is all about you. You are giving your all in service, but now it is time that you serve yourself.

You are a victor, not a victim

"The first and best victory is to conquer yourself." –
Plato

It is easy to look at your role as caregiver and claim that it is the most horrible thing that has ever happened to you and your family. You could get caught up in the downward spiral of the disease and think only of how life will change. You could take account of all the time, work, and resources you will need to put in to help out this person who is near and dear to you.

But let me frank and clear. Your position and the interpretation of what you are going through is one of the greatest powers you have over this. So do not squander this golden opportunity. I can understand how you feel. I have been at many a pity party, and I allowed it to rob me of so much love, joy, and peace. I am not a victim, and I refused to let dementia take me without a fight. I chose joy. I fight for peace. Yes, it will be hard to do all this work, but I know that my divine Creator has granted me wisdom and strength. He made provision to make sure that there was plenty of help and resources out there that could step up and partner with me. I had as much help as I requested. And based on where I was physically, financially, and emotionally, I utilized all the help that I could. I had to make the conscious declaration that I was not going to let this disease take one more day from me. I implore you to fight and to not let the disease take one more day away of you. Rise above and take your joy and never give it up without a good fight.

The work is not as important as the relationship
"It's not where you are in life, it's who you have by your side that matters." – Unknown

I will not kid you and have you think that reading this book will make the journey a cakewalk, but what I am offering you is a glimpse of hope. You are not alone. You have many around the globe who are walking through the same problems. I give you high praise for your valiant effort to toe the line and place yourself in harm's way for the sake of the person that you love. There is no higher sacrifice than that of a person willing to lay down their live for another.

I must declare that this work can be backbreaking and that there will be days that you will work yourself down to the bone. It is exhausting and depleting of all the valuable energy that you possess. Yet, each day you must rise, press on, and keep going. Love drives what you do and the level of compassion that you work with.

I want to encourage you to take a step back and see the level of work that you are doing and then compare that to the quality of the relationship you have with your loved one. Is it healthy? Is it balanced? Is it thriving? What could you do to make it better? The work you do is important, but it should never take priority or starve you from having a healthy relationship. Now, I know that because of the depleted memory and limited skills your loved one may still possess, it may be very difficult to keep a healthy relationship. I get that. But you have to be clear and real in working within the parameters that you have left. The relationship may not be great and stellar, but it can still be good. If it cannot be totally good, the fight for at least good moments throughout your day is still feasible. Do not let the disease kill the joy that can exist for you as you lift your heart to a position of highest love and care.

Chapter 15 - Boundaries and Limitations

"The best environment in which to awaken, to heal, and to grow is one of complete freedom and total safety." – Dan Brule

This is an important section if you have a loved one in your home, and they begin to show signs of difficulty with walking or sight. It is very common for dementia to diminish sight. A person can go from normal sight to a loss of peripheral vision making it so that they have what is also call tunnel vision. Based on the preexisting eye condition, blood pressure, and other health factors, along with the natural progression of dementia, this could transition very quickly for them. It is important to make sure they get a regular eye check-up, along with general and neurological checkups. With that said, it is important to understand the rapid transition in vision and the declining memory and cognitive function of your loved one and how this will change how you assist them with mobility and boundaries.

Home modification

"Don't be afraid of change, because it is leading you to a new beginning." – Joyce Meyer

You will want to treat their living environment like you would for a newborn coming to your home. You have to set up boundaries for them to keep them safe. For a child, you would make sure that you took every measure to ensure that they would not fall or roll off from where you placed them. If they were crawling, you would make sure the environment was clean and clear of thing they could pick up and place in their mouth. You would remove any object that could cut, pinch, burn, freeze, or shock them. For people living with dementia, you have to do much of the same. You have to consider that they will have some faculty of when they were active and functional, and that they will forget their limitations. To aid them, I would suggest getting rails. You will want to invest in putting in waist height rails all over you home. If you do not have the means or resources to do that, then consider arranging the furniture so that it creates a path that holds them up and guides them to their common destinations. For many, this proves to be the best method. It gives them a sense of support and it preserves their dignity. Moreover, using your furniture is less expensive than investing in hand rails all over your home.

Experiments are conducted on the various types of walkers and walking assistance devices that people with dementia use. Some of the parameters of walkers being tested are: balance, leg strength, injuries, upper body strength, vision type, and hearing capability. What researchers found is that if the user had good eyesight and good equilibrium, they did quite well with a walker, cane, or quad walker with wheels. The upper body strength made a slight difference. However, with a person with memory impairment, confusion would set in on how, when, and why they should use the walker effectively. Some would use it for a moment and then forget they were supposed to use it. They might then attempt to walk without it and fall. It is suggested that walkers and cane are unnecessary in the home. However, whenever they are out, such on a sidewalk, mall, or store it is okay for them to have the aid of these devices with monitoring. The risk is very high of them falling, so to avoid and assist, you must stay observant.

Also, you may want to consider installing high release latches on doors that you can operate from both sides of the door that prevent your loved one from entering or exiting an area without your knowledge. There are also devices that you can install into a keypad lock on any door where you have to enter a code to turn the door handle. Another suggestion to add to your home is Wi-Fi cameras that allow you to monitor your house remotely. Mainly, I want you to think in terms of creating a safe zone for your loved one where they have the freedom to move, but that also has limits that keep them from harming themselves. This will also give you more peace.

❖Chapter 15 - Boundaries and Limitations❖

Chapter 16 - Assisted Living and Nursing Homes

"Always tell someone how you feel, because opportunities are lost in the blink of an eye, but regret can last a lifetime." – Unknown

When you get to the point of thinking you need help, you are well past the level of help you need. It proved to be a hard test of the soul when I got to the point of thinking about placing my sister in a nursing home. I had heard so many horror stories about nursing homes and I did not want to allow my sister to be in one. I felt like I was failing her. I feared what could happen to her in her current state. I did not want her to be neglected or abused. However, my sister's condition worsened to a level that was beyond my level of understanding and ability to safely support. My help and resources were dwindling, and my energy was fading. A decision was required, but I had to examine my heart for the right reason to move her. I did not want to move her because I was trying to get rid of her. I did not want to move her because I was angry about the situation or what it had done to our family dynamics.

I was looking for the answer to a hard question: was it better to give her or myself the right level of care? You see, I was blindly giving up my health to make sure she had care. I did not see how bad it had become. My body ached all the time, and my stress level stayed high. I was frustrated by all that happened to me, and it started to take away the best part of my spirit. My sister's seizures were the thing that sealed my decision. I could handle her lack of memory and periodic rough demeanor. I could handle her lack of coordination and proclivity to mess-making. I could handle her hygiene issues. But when I saw her body buckle under the strain of the seizure, my heart just sank. I had to do something, but what? I was lost and had to reach out for help.

After getting good council, I knew the humane thing was to get her into a nice nursing home after I got her seizures stabilized. I found a nice place, and she seemed to be comfortable there physically. However, in her mind, it was not home. She wanted the familiarity and comfort of home. Every day that I went to see her she would ask when I was going to take her back home. Every day, and even in the night, she would wander the halls and check every door and look for a way to escape so she could get back home.

I knew she was safe and receiving excellent care. I went to see her every other day. I wanted her to know that she was not alone. As a caregiver, I want to convey to you that caring is not just about the daily duties, but it is also about the relationship you have with your loved one. You have to really, objectively look at your personal situation to determine if assisted living or a nursing home is better for your loved one, as well as for yourself. To care is no easy task, and the cycles are long and tedious. If you are not careful, it will take something good and precious from you each and every day. You have to weigh some factors to see if it is right for your case to transition your loved one to a nursing home.

As a recommendation, when you do move them, try to pick the place based on some good recommendation. Not all nursing homes are the same. Go and examine the place and the staff. You want to pick a place that has open visitation. The reason is because you want to visit intentionally at a non-scheduled time. You want to see how they treat your loved ones at various times of the day. I would also recommend getting to know all the staff by name and make sure they know you. Also, pick a place where you can customize the room decor. You want a place that lets you put up pictures and air fresheners that remind your loved one of how home looked and smelled. You will also want to get to know the activities director. Find out what types of activities they offer and how frequent. Let them know what your loved one enjoys doing.

Another issue you will want to address is your power of attorney concerning your loved one's wishes on DNR orders, feeding tubes, and any other heroic acts required to keep them alive in the event of a crisis. You want to keep them comfortable and thriving, but you will want to make sure you are not putting your loved one through extra trauma just to prolong their life. There is a point where medical care can become dehumanizing and insensitive to patient needs and to the needs of the family. In my sister's case, I had to get a court order for a DNR request and feeding tube restrictions. Based on her MRI scans, my sister's brain had severely deteriorated. Her body only functioned off of her cerebral cortex, which was basic body function. To try to prolong her life had become fruitless. But the point that I want to make here is that no matter where you place your loved one, it will not be a small decision to make. It will be a vital one. Know that you have rights and are entitled to a quality of care. To ensure that quality, you will have to stay engaged and involved. But overall, it will be better for you as a caregiver, because now you have help to carry out your tough acts of care.

Chapter 17 - The Long Goodbye

"Stories have to be told, or they die, and when they die, we can't remember who we are or why we're here." – Sue Monk Kidd, The Secret Life of Bees

This section is one of the hardest for me to write and probably for you to read. It means that there are some facts that you will have to come to terms. No one likes saying goodbye to someone they love. It seems so surreal and permanent. But I would be remiss if I did not tell you the truth. Dementia has been called the "Long Goodbye" because you see parts of your loved one drift away daily until there is nothing left. There is a level of grieving that exists that is so heavy and so painful. If you are intentional to surround yourself with the right people and work through your emotions, you can then have a means to get through the pain.

Declining health

"Your vision will become clear only when you look into your heart. Who looks inside, awakens." – Carl Jung

There is no cure to dementia. That sucks. But I have to drive this home. If your loved one is early in the stages, cherish that time and make the very best of every memory you have of them. If you are fighting to find a cure, stay strong in the fight. I have not given up hope that a cure will come. But as of today, there have been no concrete developments. Even so, I shall stay engaged until something of value is produced. With that said, I must prepare you for the slow-moving storm that is coming your way. This storm will do its best to harm your spirit and dash your hopes. The storm will bring pain that will slowly deteriorate anything that is solid and stable in your life. The storm has the potential to make you feel downright defeated. The captain of a ship knows that it is fruitless to pray, cry, or demand that the storm goes away. A storm will do what it needs to do. It will blow until it is done. But a good captain knows that the right thing to do is not to change the storm, but to change their sails. You cannot stop the storm, but you can use the energy of the storm to move you to a better place.

What I am trying to imply is that for the sake of your health as a caregiver, you have to realize death is something your loved one will have to go through, and you have to go through it with them. You can choose to walk in defeat, or you can choose to snatch victory from the jaws of defeat. You can choose to fight for their dignity, fight for their spirit, fight for their comfort, and fight for their peace of mind. Fight so that they are never treated less than human. Fight to make sure anyone who sees them knows that this person is meaningful and valued. Fight to make sure their pain is minimum. Fight to make sure their wishes are honored and fight to make sure all of their affairs are in order. Fight to make sure the world knows that your loved one lived, loved, and mattered.

Hospice care

"...We could never learn to be brave and patient if there were only joys in the world..." - Helen Keller

Because of the nature of this disease, pieces of your loved one will be lost each day. If engage in care and you help meet day to day needs, you will see subtle changes over time. You will see an up and down progression each and every day. This is where it gets painful to watch someone you love deteriorate, and die every day. And when I say die, I do mean to die. The memory of their life is stripped away. Things they used to do, they no longer can do. Their personality and the best parts of them are gone to never be seen again.

How do you cope with this? Well, what helped me is never committing to bottle up what I was experiencing. I was experiencing grief each and every day of the care process. It is bad enough when you lose someone suddenly, let alone knowing it is coming from a long way out. However, I have learned through my involvement with other grief counseling sessions that it is extremely healthy and therapeutic to talk, express, journal, write poems, tell stories, and tell friends about how you feel. The longer and deeper you keep it inside, the harder the grieving process will be.

During the last three months of my sister's life, I had to seek the help of hospice care. The group that I brought in helped take a load off physically and mentally with what I had to address with caring for my sister. I was out of my depth when it came to walking with someone for the last mile of their life. I did not know what to look for or what to expect. The team that helped me out brought in a highly skilled nurse as well as a spiritual advisor. The nurse talked to me every other day and gave me a play by play explanation of what my sister's body was going through and the level of pain she was experiencing. The nurse helped me count down the days and allowed for the family and me to have the time we needed to say goodbye. Even though my sister could not hear or understand what we were saying to her, hospice still provided the help and insight we needed to go gradually through this transition.   On a spiritual level, they were equally valuable as well. My sister was a woman true to her faith. When she was in her stable mind, she loved to share her faith and lived out what it means. The person from hospice would come and pray with her and sang old church hymns to her. They were doing their best to reassure her that her faith was true and gave her the comfort she needed as she went the last leg of her journey. I am so thankful to them for their faithful service. Even after her passing, they still provided follow-up to see how we were doing and to assess if we had any needs or anything to express. That made a huge difference in dealing with the passing and the pain.

Do not walk through this alone
"Walking with a friend in the dark is better than walking alone in the light." – Helen Keller

Over my short life, I have walked through a lot of loss. I have lost both of my parents. My dad died at an early age and my mom died at a crucial time in my life; I lost a brother that I was close to; I lost a sister, who I never had a chance to meet, who died not too long before I was born. I have lost friends and co-workers. Some of those were close personal friends and others were acquaintances. Of all these experiences, there was one common thread that I noticed that got me through the grieving. The first thing to note was that I chose to be vocal about how I was feeling. I had to be real with my expressions, and I had to leave room to say what was on my mind, without having someone edit my pain. I found that grief is a hallway, one with a start and finish. The pain and loss do not go away, but as you walk through that hall, and pour out that grief, the weight of that grief becomes less and less. My expression of pain and frustration acted as a pressure valve. The situation allowed me room to blow off steam.

The other thing that helped me through my pain and grief of the disease and my sister's passing was my passion for becoming thankful in my outlook and expressions. My attitude took a shift over a long period, what I found is that the more expressions of thanksgiving I made, the better my grieving process went. I found myself thanking everyone for every little thing that they did for me. I thank the clerk that processes my order at the bank. I thank the server that provides my food. I thanked the nurses that provided care while my sister was in the hospital. I thanked the doctors and staff. I thank family, friends and co-workers at every turn that I can. I would encourage any of you to develop an attitude of thankfulness and gratitude. It will give you the power to overcome and the strength to deal with the grief you have to walk through. And when I say "walk through," I do mean walk through. Do not try to dodge it, but take into account the full experience of death. You need to express your emotions.

That leads me to the third and most important healing process: be deliberate and willing to change and enhance your surroundings. What I mean by that is the people you surround yourself with. Find people you understand and that can relate to what you are going through. Find people who have lived through your trials. Find people who are strong, loving, and caring. When you are going through tough times, you will need a shoulder to cry on and a hand to lift you up. You will need a word of wisdom and encouragement. You will need a sound ear that will listen to you. Overall, you are going to need someone, whether you believe it or not. You can choose to go it alone, or you can choose to seek the help of others. I have tried it both ways, and the way that has helped me the most in the time of need was through the help of others.

Plan ahead
"The secret to getting ahead is getting started." – Mark Twain

We make plans all the time for things we want to do in the future. We plan for vacations, and we plan for our career. We plan our meals, and if we are attending school, we plan what type of classes we will take. We plan for the dream house we want, and we think about how to get the fancy car we always dreamed about. Planning is empowering and liberating. When we plan, especially about things that we want to do, there is an air of excitement.   Sometimes we can hardly contain ourselves for what is yet to come. Sometimes, the better we plan, the less anxiety we have about what is coming.

So if we can plan for something that we desire to do, and find that it empowers us and helps reduce our stress, then it will be logical to experience some of the same feelings when planning for things that we do not exactly love. When it comes to caring for loved ones, there are going to be some tough decisions, and some that are even life changing. When it comes to care, it is very helpful to talk about your plan. If you can plan with other helpers, then that would help distribute the load. Even if you are going it alone, it is still a great idea to write out your plans.

You should record your plan for care in regards to your role and the entire task that you have to perform. Record your strengths and limitations. Record the names and roles of others involved in the care process. Record the names of doctors and insurance information. Include in your plan the doctor suggested treatment plan. You will also want to document the progression of care as your loved one's health declines. Record what their wishes are and how they can be carried out.

The advantage to writing this down is that it gives you a play-by-play look at upcoming tasks. It also gives you a visual reference on what is working and what is not, and how to best modify it. Another advantage is that it takes a load off your mind that if you cannot carry out your duties, there will be someone who can pick up your plan and carry on where you left off. The plan will also function as a communication tool for any interested party, especially when it comes to final plans and wishes. I have seen so many people go to battle simply because there were too many people stepping in at the last minute and imposing plans and wishes that were not in compliance with the will of the one in need of care. This will always result in a major conflict. Simply put, to reduce the stress, be diligent to sit down and write a plan, even if it is not pretty or perfect. It will be a living document. You will be changing it from time to time. But the important thing is that you do some form of organized planning.

Know your rights
"Be suborn about your goals, and flexible about your methods." – Unknown

You want to make sure that your loved one is getting the best in care, whether it is in your home or a care facility. You want them to be safe and treated like a human being. You want dignity to be a high priority. There are a few legal entities to consider when considering the care you and a nursing home will give your loved one. These will be discussed next and include: the federal government, the state agencies, the local court systems, the hospital, the nursing home, and the family.

The Federal Government

"Your value does not decrease based on someone's inability to see your worth." – Unknown

The feds have a role they must play when it comes to care. They generate laws and rules regarding funding, support, and medical research related to care. I would say, at the forefront, that what you need and should be demanding from your government is federal dollars to support research. They should be finding every available resource to support studies and development of medicines and cures. I want an army of people engaged with every senator and lawmaker on the subject of elder care and especially dementia research. There is a cure on the horizon. We must pull our resources and fight until the cure is brought home. If we can rally and fight in wars around the globe to stop terror, we can at least spend a fraction of that to fight on our home front and end terror in the minds of the ones that we love. Now that is a dollar well spent.

As a US citizen, you also have a right to request disability support. This is funding that is granted to help those who are in need. It is not a lot of money, but it is still available to help meet some needs. Also, if your loved one needs it, make sure they apply for Medicare part A and B medical insurance. Even if your loved one is young, they still may be eligible for this support. My experience is that practically everyone who applies is initially denied. However, even if you were working closely with doctors and neurologists, it would be in your best interest to contact your local elder law attorney and utilize their assistance, especially if they have experience with federal disability cases. This dramatically increases your odds of getting your case approve. Bear in mind that there will be legal fees. However, you can arrange with your SSI agent to get the fees paid out of the disability agreement once the case is settled.

The state agencies
"Progress is impossible without change, and those who cannot change their minds cannot change anything." – George Bernard Shaw

Just like the federal government, you must hold your local governments feet to the fire in the war on dementia. I want you to pay close attention to elections and rally events taking place. I want you to attend nominee's rallies and go to their websites, Facebook pages, and Twitter accounts and start asking all the questions that you can by way of how much support they are willing to give and how committed they are when it comes to research and development for a cure for dementia. Ask what their views are on elder support and care. If they have responded and given a positive answer, then hit their opponent with the same question. Make it clear this is addressed. If not addressed, the weight of this coming epidemic is enough to bankrupt your local state due to how much it will cost to provide long-term care. If we can fight for a cure and set up prevention, we can help sustain our state's resources.

We have to push our states to get into gear by making sure there are enough nursing homes to accommodate the rapid growing needs for the next 20 years. We need to push our state to make sure that there are trained workers who are well versed in caring for the needs of those with dementia. We cannot wait on this. We have to act now.

If you have any other ideas that I may have missed, please send me an email or post your comments on what we can do on *CourageousCaregiver.org*. Together we can make a huge difference.

The local court systems

"You may encounter many defeats, but you must not be defeated." – Maya Angelou

The local court level is there to safeguard the rights of your loved one. They are there to assist you with providing care within the confines of the law. They can help with granting power of attorney, guardianship, and conservatorship over assets. They are also helpful with legal decisions related to the end of life care. Bear in mind that they will want to make sure the rights of your loved one are completely protected. So they will assign a guardian ad lithium to review the case and any requests you may make regarding assets and health. No matter what you ask or may need from them, it is very important that you keep good detailed records and can present your requests and concerns in writing. The judge has to make decisions based on the law and evidence presented. It is your goal to provide as much detail as possible so they can make a good legal decision.

The hospital
"They may forget your name, but they will never forget how you made them feel." – Maya Angelou

The role that hospitals play when it comes to the care of your loved one is emergency triage care and advanced testing, along with extensive care, especially related to aftercare from surgery. The things that go on in a hospital are amazing, and the way they provide care has advanced over the years. Especially at the student-based learning hospitals. I appreciate the research and developments that have taken place over the past ten years. If it were not for that work, we would not know as much as we do about the disease or how to treat it.

As good as hospitals are, there is still a lot of room for improvement. But the improvement must first come from out awareness of the rights we have as patients. First of all, the loved one under your care has rights. You must be diligent and persistent in asking what their wishes are. Do your very best to honor what you can and develop a happy medium for that which you have difficulty fulfilling

With dementia, there will be various reasons your loved one may have to go through a hospital stay. Many dementia patients in the later stages will be prone to infections and pneumonia. If it gets bad enough, they will have to be treated with strong antibiotics. With my sister's Lewy-Bodies Dementia, she developed rabdo-miloasis, which is a hardening of the muscles due to the body not passing fluids to major muscle groups. During the hospital stay, I realized that my sister was in her last stages of dementia, and I, as well as other family members, did not want any heroics or extreme measures to try to prolong her life. The hospital either had to get it in writing from the patient or a power of attorney that indicated what the patient wishes were. In my case, I only had basic guardianship. So I had to go to probate court and petition to have a DNR and a "no intubation indicator" placed on her chart to keep them from having to institute hospital policy to try to sustain her life. This is a difficult matter many families have to face. You have to know your loved one's wishes, and you have fight to ensure their support.

You have to understand that hospitals are there to assist doctors and nursing homes with extreme cases. The methods that they use to help are extensive and expensive. Make sure to ask a lot of questions about the level of coverage. Make sure to fill out all privacy forms and make sure to address all legal authorization forms. If you are at the point where you need hospice service, make sure to understand what level of service they are going to provide in conjunction to what service you will be needing. Not all hospice care services are the same, so you therefore must make sure you clearly understand what they will be doing and go as far to ask how much it will cost. That service is not free, and if you are not able to afford it, it may be a huge sticker shock. As long as you have filled out the HIPPA form, you do have a right to know what is going on, and you have the right to refuse services that you do not agree to or support. Do not allow the medical team to intimidate you because you may be in a vulnerable state of mind.

They have a policy and procedure they have to follow, but that does not mean that it agrees with your values, plans, or beliefs.

The nursing home
"I do not understand the mystery of grace, only that it meets us where we are but does not leave us where we are found." – Anne Lamott

If you have done your homework and review and interview your nursing home and its ratings, conditions, and procedures, you will find that a nursing home is a wonderful place for your loved one. You want a place where you have freedom of access 24/7. Some do not offer that. Some limit visitation for the sake of keeping the environment calm for the patient. If you feel like you are having restricted access to your loved one, then that should be a sign of concern. I am not saying that nursing homes are deliberate in abusing patients, but a good nursing home will bend over backward to make sure that the doors are open and that everything is exposed.

Not all nursing homes are the same. The standards could be all over the chart. Also, when you compare it to your personal living condition, their standard may be how you keep your home. But with that said, I want you to know that your loved one does not have to settle being in one that feels and projects itself as a garbage hole. There are some that are out there that should have their doors shut. I do not want you responding out of desperation to find one at the last minute and end up with what is left over. So, please do your homework, and make a list of three or four in your area that measure up to the standard you want well before you get to the point of really having to place your loved one in a nursing home.

On your visit to the nursing homes, look for signs of life. First of all, check to see if the receptionist greets and smiles at you. Some places do not even have a reception. A good place will have a trained and caring gatekeeper. Once you are in the door, sniff the air. Does it smell of cleanliness or as if someone had been cleaning or does it reek of old musk? That smell is an indicator of how much time and attention they put on each patient. Ask about activities: how often are they offered and what type do they offer. Ask if there are any limitations on participating. Check out the cafeteria. How is the food? If the food is poor in taste and quality, are you allowed to bring in food for your loved one from time to time? Do they have a trained dietitian? Also, ask if you have the right to check your loved one out for a visit, just in case you want to take them out for a walk or to visit their local worship center?

Based on the condition of your loved one, many nursing homes have to follow some of the same procedure as a hospital as to how they administer care. Especially if they are a Medicaid level nursing home. This means that you have to address all the paperwork the same. You must have the means to address all medical decisions. Finally, do not give the nursing home the free reign to make a decision about care and treatment unless it is authorized by yourself.

Family

"The love in our family flows strong and deep, leaving us memories to treasure and keep." – Unknown

If you have a strong and loving family, that could make all the difference in the world. I have two lovely sisters that helped me out in a huge way—my oldest sister, Loraine, and my baby sister, Ora. They were angels in backing me up with care in areas that I could not perform, or they simply stepped in when I was worn out. In a way, they saved my life and made the workload a lot lighter. However, as great as they were, there were areas that came up while we were caring for our other sister that became a concern. Each person has a different level of care they would provide, based on their point of view. This was not necessarily a bad thing, but we did not always agree on everything. It is all right to disagree, but it has to be done in a cooperative manner. Because of my sister's wishes and the role I played, everyone knew that I had the final word in any debate.

One area where we came in conflict was on the issue of medication. I had to stay apprised of what my sister was taking, and I had to examine the results we were getting. There were times that other family members visited my sister at the hospital, and they did not agree with what was being issued. They insisted to the hospital staff that the medication be changed. It was a good thing that I had legal guardianship over the case, because that granted me authority over the medical care. I had to get it placed on my sister's chart to make sure that all medical decisions and changes were run through me before a change was granted. I also had to limit how much information was being granted related to her medical status. The danger with the flow of information was that once it got out, it would spread like wildfire and then eventually come back to me in a form very different than when it went out. So I had to make the conscious decision to cut off or limit what was being told about my sister's current state.

You need to know that you have a right to lead and right to love. You will find that as you engage in care and as things get rough, people will talk a mean game about how they will be there for you, but in many cases, when the going gets tough, the crowd diminishes. They will show up again in the final hour, but not when the heavy lifting is needed. As a caregiver, you will need to make a tough and hard decision. You have earned the right to make those decisions. Make them based on the level of care you have put in and on the level of love that you have for your loved one. Be free in your thinking and be free in your expression of love. Most of all, do not second-guess yourself to appease the feeling of others that are not directly involved.

Caregiver contingency plan
"Failing to plan is planning to fail." – Unknown

As a caregiver, it is easy to get engrossed in the work you are doing and the level of support you have to provide. However, it is extremely important to develop a contingency plan just in case you are unable to fulfill your duties. Please allow me to share a story of one of the families I counseled.   In this case, there was a husband and wife who loved and cared for each other. When the wife was in her late 40s, she started to show signs of early onset dementia. The husband's love for his wife was so great that he stepped up his level of care to the point where he could manage to keep her disease a secret to their friends and even their adult children. As time went on, the husband got ill to the point of death. After he had passed away, the adult children came back to help their mom put together the arrangements. This is when they first discovered how bad off their mom was. The dad did not leave a will or written plan on how to address the needs of his wife and none of the children had a clue as to what they could do to take care of their mother.

You need to take time to identify who could be best qualified to support in your absence. You then will have to sit down and talk with your substitute about the level of backup support that would be required. At that point, work with them to adjust the plan so that it can meet both of your needs. Give them room to decline the responsibility. That way, if they feel they cannot do it, you can then develop other resources. Another resource to consider is a nursing home. As stated above, do your homework. Find out your top three facilities. Make sure your research gets recorded in your written plan. Once you have your plan written, you can then pick a few trusted relatives and friends to share that information with. That way, if something happens, you at least can have the peace of mind that someone has seen your plan, and then someone can step up and find it and execute it.

Hire care
"Individually we are one drop. Together we're an ocean." – Unknown

There is an epidemic in our nation. We have a massive amount of baby boomers retiring and needing care. Many people will end up in nursing homes. This is leading to a huge shortage of nursing homes across this nation. They are working feverishly to build new places. However, it cannot keep up with the rising demand. Many people are looking into hiring at home care. There are many agencies out there, but not all places are alike. So, first of all, I would start with a couple of resources. First I would get on the web and do a search for "senior care at home." This will produce a list of agencies that could potentially help. One place that I have been seeing advertise on TV is "Home Instead Senior Care." They give a list of services that they provide, and you can pick and choose what you would have them come in and do based on your needs. One cool service that I saw that they offered is training on how to care for your loved one with dementia. They will send someone to your home, and they will do an assessment of your care needs and then based on the assessment, they can walk you through a series of care techniques that would work best for your loved one with Alzheimer's or dementia. Either way, you have help available. Do not hesitate to make that call. Make sure to go to *CourageousCaregiver.org* to check out my listing of recommended places that could provide help and services as well.

Set up daycare

"If you truly love someone, then the only thing you want for them is to be happy … Even if it's not with you." – Lauren

There can never be enough adult day cares to go around if they are anything like the one I had. In Auburn Hills, Michigan, there is a place that is a slice right out of heaven, The Adult Quality of Life Center.

They treated each person as if they were family. Jackie, the director, was very passionate about the care and love she gave to each person that entered her doors. That place and the workers were gems. I highly recommend that you look into availability in your area. Review offerings and take the time to give it a walk-through visit. You will want to see what they do with the participants in the morning as well as the afternoon. You will want to see it when other patients are present. You want to see how the staff relates to and interacts with each person under their care. Make a list of pros and cons and then make sure to review this list against other daycare facilities in your area.

Grief and lifestyle change
"Some people come into our life and quickly go. Some stay for a while and leave footprints on our hearts and us never, ever the same." – C. C. Scott

I am not going to kid you. Caring for someone with dementia is a task loaded with grief. It is something that you cannot escape. Since you cannot escape it, then you had better learn how best to go through it. First of all, be real and honest with yourself about the fact that your life, and the life of your loved one, will change. It will get more and more difficult every day. You will see their body every day, but each day you will see pieces of them fall away. It is painful to watch. I know I have said this before, but I want to bring this point home. One of my best allies was the power of thanksgiving. I had to develop a high level of gratitude for every minute detail of my life. This raised my sense of awareness, and it enabled me to draw in what I needed to give me perspective and strength to face my loss. It is okay to stay hopeful about your loved one getting better, but to go along with that is cherishing every moment of their life and how their life mattered. By holding to that love, no matter where the transition takes you, you can face it with a thankful heart and a clear conscious.

Practicing the presence of God

"No matter where you go, you carry the presence of God. So shine brightly, for you may be the only light they may every get a chance to see." – Cal Garcia

I have spent a lot of time nurturing and developing my faith. There are things that I have learned from my faith that have given me the skills to navigate the journey of life. Like a ship at sea, I am in motion, and the sea is ever changing. Some days, the seas are calm, and other days the wind is strong and steady. Other days the waves are fierce, and the storm rages. I cannot stop the sea from being the sea, but I can choose to change my sail. By changing my sail, I can get from life all that it has to offer and I get to travel to places and meet people and not allow the condition of the sea to hinder. That same philosophy has taken me on some fantastic journeys and taught me so much. Of all that I learned, I want to share two things, that will be of value to you like it was for me in my trials I faced when caring for my sister: carry the presence of the kingdom into any situation and do not let other things dim your light.

Carrying the presence of the kingdom into any situation

"When you enter God's presence with praise, He enters your circumstances with power." – Unknown

My faith tells me that there is more to life than what I presently see. My faith tells me that there is a Creator of all of this. Now, at this point, I am not proselytizing, but I am sharing a little about how faith has aided me to deliver the best in care as well as face some hard moments. Each day I grow in my faith, I became more aware and engaged in life. Each day I spend exploring my faith, I draw more of that essence into my being which then grants me the means to radiate that essence into every place I go and to everyone I encounter. My love for my Creator has in turn centered a high amount of love that I was able to lavish upon my sister. That love allowed me to be at peace and to show patience. Just like my Creator granted me patience in my development, He also enabled me to show powerful patience and peace to others. I found that there was no limit to the places or the people I could bless by simply being all that I could be in my faith.

Do not let other things dim the light

"Don't let someone dim your light simply because it is shining in their eyes." – Unknown

Darkness and light cannot co-exist. Light a small match in a dark room, and watch the darkness immediately rush away. My faith has called me to be a shining light in a dark world. The world that I had been called to deal with was the mind of my sister. She felt unsure of herself and alone. So each day I had to bring the refreshing light of trust and reassurance. I had to bring presence and love. I was able to help her feel happy and confident. This disease took a lot from my sister. However, I did not allow it to take anything without a strong fight. Where she could not fight, I stood and fought in her place. Through the illumination of love, I was able to brighten her day and usher in a calming outlook.

Chapter 18 – What's Next

"Start by doing what's necessary; then do what's possible, and suddenly you are doing the impossible." – Francis of Assisi

Before I bring this book to a close, I wanted to share with you some things that I have experienced during this writing project. I felt so blessed to serve, and I am so excited by this experience. I know that this writing project has saved my life. I learned a lot and gained some new friends along the way. Out of this writing was birthed a few other projects that are in the works. Also, I really would love for you to get yourself signed up for my email Newsletter, so I can keep you apprised of future development.

What is on the horizon?

"If it doesn't challenge you, it doesn't change you." – Fred Devito

I also want to promote another project that my friend clued me in on. There is a need of resources for those who are homebound by their care, but who also still want to have a job. So I am developing a book and training guide and video series to help those that are at home set up a home-based business. There are a lot of opportunities out there, and it is way easier than you think to develop something that could work for you and your situation. Keep checking the website and watch for it to come out soon.

DVD and online training videos for support groups

"Life challenges are not supposed to paralyze you; they're supposed to help you discover who you are." – Bernice Johnson Reagan

I had some other fans, who I am eternally grateful for, ask me to describe some of the things I had to do to take care of my sister. I have told so many stories, over and over again. So someone suggested that I record some of my conversations and make a DVD that they could have. I initially thought it was way too much work, but in reality, that was a smart idea. So I am in the studios now to develop the videos. That way, when people ask, I can just tell them to check out the DVD or download one of the videos from my website. I hope you are blessed by what I am developing. If you have any questions or want to see certain topics covered in the videos, please go to *CourageousCaregiver.org* and leave a comment or drop me an email, and I will make a way for your concern to get addressed and out there.

Support group webinars

"I want to inspire people. I want someone to look at me and say, 'Because of you I didn't give up.'" – Unknown

This is one that gets the wheels spinning and the juices salivating. Years ago, I used to teach. I taught when I was with the military, I did career training on a technical level, and I did biblical training at my church. There has always been something so fulfilling about doing that. So, in conjunction with this book, I will be introducing training videos and webinars. Also, my vision is to take this one step further. Whether we believe it or not, we need each other. We may not say it outright, and there are those who have given up on humanity, but there are still those out there that care and have a passion for seeing others loved, supported, cared for and successful. So, via my website, you will see links, tools, and features coming out that will help us develop a community of friends and supporters. It will help us stay connected and support each other at the highest level.

Conclusion

"Take on risk and ride the journey called life with no regrets." - Unknown

This has been one phenomenal journey. I got to live, love, matter, and make sure that my sister's life mattered as well. I got to participate in a labor of love. I got stretched in more ways than one. I got to face down some giants in my life, and I can clearly say, that I feel like a winner. I got a chance to tell my sister's story. I got to bless some people along the way. And I got past my fears of failure and wrote something worth publishing. I am so grateful for this opportunity to serve you in this capacity.

I hope you had an eye-opening experience as to what someone with dementia faces. I hope you got a chance to see yourself in what I shared. I hope you see that you have been granted a higher and nobler purpose. Not everyone has the heart to do what you are doing. Not everyone can serve. Many can serve, but not all can soar. I hope this book gives you wings. Rise to a higher height within yourself. Take off all the limits. Love at your highest capacity.

If there is one thing I hope you can walk away with after reading this book, it is that you can hold your head up high and say that you made a difference. Moreover, I hope that you have found within yourselves the power to say "thank you." I use those words religiously. Each time my left foot touches the ground, I say to myself, or out loud if the situation permits, "thank." Then as my right foot touches the ground, I say "you." I consciously repeat that cycle over and over again, all throughout my day. You see, I have a conscious choice to look at the past or my current situation and allow my mind to interpret it in a way that says I am a loser. I could say that what I am going though can and will defeat me, or I can choose to give thanks that as bad as my life may seem, I still have life and choice, and I can do something about my circumstances. I give thanks for the life I have, and I give thanks for getting to serve my sister. I give thanks that God granted me time to connect with her. I give thanks for every life I get to impact someone else's life. I give thanks for the cure that is soon on its way. I give thanks for the amazing connections that will grow from and through the people that will read and share this book. I can truly say that the blessing is all mine.

If you noticed while reading this book, the tempo and content changed. My sister was doing pretty stable when I started this book, but she had the honor and pleasure of being promoted into her higher state of being, as she closed her eyes and drew her last breath, on June 7, 2015. My time with her helped me to confirm that her faith was intact, and that she was at peace. My heart was at peace in knowing that I gave her my best and that she brought out the best in me. I hated this journey at the beginning and now I can embrace it without the pain of grief. I still do miss her and all the time we spent together. There are time when I am cooking that I think about what she would like to eat. Of after she entered the nursing home, there was a certain route I would take to get there. I would find myself compelled to drive in that direction sometimes when I would leave work and then I would stop and catch myself. Above all, this is a deep and moving process. It caused me to grow in wisdom and expression. I give praise for the opportunity to serve her, and to now serve others. Thank you for reading and being a part of this journey.

There is a very powerful quote that was passed along to me, and I hold it near and dear: "a part of living with the disease is living." It is my heartfelt belief that life discovery happens in some of life's darkest moments simply by choosing to seek it. My friends, if you are engaging in the throes of care, trim your sails and set a course toward hope. Trust in your newfound knowledge and in your crew—the fellow supporters of this project. Know that you are not alone. I look at my personal fears as being dark, and I look at love as being light. I have made it my passion to love at the highest level and to let the light drive away all fear and darkness. I encourage you to love yourself. The way you love yourself creates a means for love to come your way, and it sets the standard for how you will be able to love. Also, know that love is like a flower. The better you take care of it, the more it grows and the brighter it gets. Love hard and let the development amaze you.

Once again, it was my pleasure to have you read my story and to help you grow in your own heart. If you think this book has helped you, I would ask that you purchase a copy and pass it along to a friend that you know that may be facing a similar issue. We are not in this alone. The more we step up now, the less damage this disease can do.

❖Chapter 18 – What's Next❖

Thanks again for all your love, prayers, and support.

REMEMBER

The Caregiver Commitment

LIVE ❖LOVE ❖ LEAVE

*As a caregiver, I commit to **LIVE** my life at its highest level and to make sure I show up for it every day and in every way.*

*I commit to **LOVE** everyone that is placed in front of me and find a way to love what I am doing in full joy.*

*I commit to live my life in such a way that it becomes legendary and contagious and I **LEAVE** a legacy that shapes the world I live in because I simply chose to stand up and do something about it.*

About the Author:

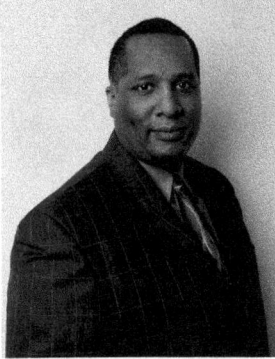

Curtis Walker is a first-time author and lover and liver of life. He was born in Pontiac, Michigan and lived in Michigan for most of his life. He is married to Tamara, and they have two adult children, Jonathan and Lina. He spent nine years in the U. S. Marine Reserves from 1992 to 2003. He is a graduate of the University of Phoenix with a B. S. in Information Technology. He is the sole brother of four older sisters and very proud of it. He loves his family and encourages them daily. He is engaged in his community and world relief missions. Stay plugged in and keep your eyes open for other great books like this one to come out shortly.